# Responsible Opioid Prescribing™

## A CLINICIAN'S GUIDE

**SECOND EDITION
REVISED AND EXPANDED**

Scott M. Fishman, MD

*This accredited Continuing Medical Education (CME) activity is jointly sponsored by:*

  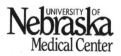

Published by Waterford Life Sciences, Washington, DC
Tel: 202-299-0600 | Email: jhorwitz@waterfordls.com
Cover and Book Design: Gretchen Maxwell, GLM Design

**Responsible Opioid Prescribing**™ is a trademark of the Federation of State
Medical Boards Research and Education Foundation

This edition of **Responsible Opioid Prescribing**™ A Clinician's Guide
is published with support from the Substance Abuse and Mental
Health Services Administration, U.S. Department of Health and
Human Services.

## Target Audience

This activity is intended for physicians, dentists, podiatrists, nurse practitioners, physician assistants, and other health professionals who prescribe opioids in their clinical practice.

## Statement of Need

Opioid analgesics have become controversial drugs that are widely used for the management of moderate to severe pain, but are also widely abused and diverted for non-medical purposes. Opioids are among the most prescribed drug classes in the United States, and the science supporting their effectiveness for chronic pain has remained weak, while evidence reflecting the substantial problem of prescription drug abuse has become stronger. There is inadequate knowledge among many prescribers about pain management, about the risks associated with the use of opioid drugs, and particularly about the risk of addiction. There is also evidence that prescribers' decisions about opioid prescribing have been influenced by their lack of knowledge about the laws and regulations that govern the prescribing of these drugs. The current environment of widespread under-treatment of pain alongside rampant prescription drug abuse highlights the need to educate prescribers about risk management when treating pain with opioid analgesic drugs.

This CME activity is designed to improve the knowledge of practicing physicians and other prescribers about the laws and regulations that govern the prescribing of opioid analgesics for pain control. It is specifically aimed at helping physicians and other prescribers learn the steps they can take to develop a risk management-oriented approach to pain management. It will help clinicians who prescribe opioids understand the expectations of medical boards and other regulators, particularly concerning comprehensive and ongoing risk management. It will also inform clinicians about their parallel responsibility to treat patients with pain—whether with opioid or non-opioid therapies—while minimizing the risk to their patients, and to society at large, of prescription drug abuse.

# ABMS Compentencies Covered in This Activity

This CME activity has been designed to promote all six of the core competencies for quality patient care promulgated by the American Board of Medical Specialties:

- **Professionalism**—Demonstrate a commitment to carrying out professional responsibilities, adherence to ethical principles and sensitivity to diverse patient populations.
- **Patient Care and Procedural Skills**—Provide care that is compassionate, appropriate and effective treatment for health problems and to promote health.
- **Medical Knowledge**—Demonstrate knowledge about established and evolving biomedical, clinical and cognate sciences and their application in patient care.
- **Practice-based Learning and Improvement**—Able to investigate and evaluate their patient care practices, appraise and assimilate scientific evidence and improve their practice of medicine.
- **Interpersonal and Communication Skills**—Demonstrate skills that result in effective information exchange and teaming with patients, their families and professional associates (e.g. fostering a therapeutic relationship that is ethically sound, uses effective listening skills with non-verbal and verbal communication; working as both a team member and at times as a leader).
- **Systems-Based Practice**—Demonstrate awareness of and responsibility to larger context and systems of healthcare. Be able to call on system resources to provide optimal care (e.g. coordinating care across sites or serving as the primary case manager when care involves multiple specialties, professions or sites).

## Learning Objectives

The content of this CME activity is divided into three Modules:

### MODULE 1: RISK ASSESSMENT, PATIENT SELECTION, AND TREATMENT PLANNING

At the conclusion of this activity, participants should be able to:

- Discuss current data on risks associated with long-term opioid therapy.
- Describe, screen for, and assess risk factors in patients being selected for potential opioid therapy.
- Design and employ the basic components of an effective pain treatment plan, including functional goals and a discontinuation strategy.

**MODULE 2: INITIATING, DOCUMENTING, MONITORING AND DISCONTINUING OPIOID THERAPY**

At the conclusion of this activity, participants should be able to:
- Demonstrate ability to reach clear agreements with patients about rights and responsibilities in opioid prescribing relationship.
- Practice clear documentation of prescribing history, including informed consent and progress, if any, towards functional goals.
- Differentiate among patients who have developed tolerance, physical dependence and/or addiction to opioid analgesics.
- Employ approaches manage patient being treated with opioid analgesics who exhibit behaviors that may be indicative of substance abuse, including discontinuation of opioid therapy.

**MODULE 3: MANAGING SPECIAL RISK POPULATIONS AND SITUATIONS**

At the conclusion of this activity, participants should be able to:
- Recognize special risks associated with methadone treatment for pain.
- Apply effective communication strategies for educating patients and caregivers on safe use, storage and disposal of opioid medications.
- Identify special risks of drug misuse among young people.
- Perform the current simple steps required to be in compliance with controlled substances laws and regulations.

## Accreditation Statement

This activity has been planned and implemented in accordance with the Essential Areas and Policies of the Accreditation Council for Continuing Medical Education through the joint sponsorship of The University of Nebraska Medical Center, Center for Continuing Education, the Federation of State Medical Boards Research and Education Foundation, and the Federation of State Medical Boards. The University of Nebraska Medical Center is accredited by the Accreditation Council for Continuing Medical Education to provide continuing medical education for physicians.

## Credit Designation

### PHYSICIANS

The University of Nebraska Medical Center, Center for Continuing Education designates this enduring material for a maximum of 7.25 *AMA PRA Category 1 Credits*™. Physicians should claim only the credit commensurate with the extent of their participation in the activity.

Participants will receive a certificate upon completion of each activity. Nurse practitioners, nurses and physician assistants may utilize activities that are certified by ACCME-accredited providers toward their requirement for certification and/or licensure. Other health professionals should verify whether the credit for these activities meets certification and/or licensure requirements for their discipline.

## Release Date: May 1, 2012
## Expiration Date: May 1, 2014

### Disclosure

It is the policy of the University of Nebraska Medical Center, Center for Continuing Education to ensure balance, independence, objectivity, and scientific rigor in all its sponsored educational activities. All faculty, activity planners, content reviewers, and staff participating in this activity have disclosed to the participants any significant financial interest or other relationship with manufacturer(s) of any commercial product(s)/device(s) and/or provider(s) of commercial services included in this educational activity. The intent of this disclosure is not to prevent a person with a relevant financial or other relationship from participating in the activity, but rather to provide participants with information on which they can base their own judgments. The University of Nebraska Medical Center, Center for Continuing Education has identified and resolved any and all conflicts of interest prior to the release of this activity.

### Resolution of Conflicts of Interest

In accordance with the Accreditation Council for Continuing Medical Education Standards for Commercial Support of CME, the University of Nebraska Medical Center, Center for Continuing Education has implemented mechanisms prior to the planning and implementation of this CME activity to identify and resolve conflicts of interest for all individuals in a position to control content of this CME activity.

## Faculty
**Author: Scott M. Fishman, MD**
Professor and Chief, Division of Pain Medicine
    Department of Anesthesiology and Pain Medicine
    University of California, Davis
Disclosure: No relevant financial relationships to disclose

**Medical Writer: Stephen Braun**
Disclosure: No relevant financial relationships to disclose

**Reviewer: Keith M. Olsen, PharmD, FCCP, FCCM**
Professor and Chair, The University of Nebraska Medical Center,
    College of Pharmacy
Disclosure: No relevant financial relationships to disclose

## Staff Disclosures
Neither the planners, reviewers, editors, staff, CME committee, nor other members at the University of Nebraska Medical Center, Center for Continuing Education who control content have any relevant financial relationships to disclose.

Neither the planners, reviewers, editors, staff, CME committee, nor other members of the Federation of State Medical Boards Research and Education Foundation and the Federation of State Medical Boards who control content have any relevant financial relationships to disclose.

## Unapproved Use Disclosure
The University of Nebraska Medical Center, Center for Continuing Education requires CME faculty (speakers) to disclose to the attendees when products or procedures being discussed are off-label, unlabeled, experimental, and/or investigational (not FDA approved); and any limitations on the information that is presented, such as data that are preliminary or that represent ongoing research, interim analyses, and/or unsupported opinion. Faculty in this activity may discuss information about pharmaceutical agents that is outside of U.S. Food and Drug Administration approved labeling. This information is intended solely for continuing medical education and is not intended to promote off-label use of these medications. If you have questions, contact the medical affairs department of the manufacturer for the most recent prescribing information.

## Privacy Policy

The University of Nebraska Medical Center protects the privacy of personal and other information regarding participants and educational collaborators. The University of Nebraska Medical Center will not release personally identifiable information to a third party without the individual's consent, except such information as is required for reporting purposes to the Accreditation Council for Continuing Medical Education. The University of Nebraska Medical Center maintains physical, electronic, and procedural safeguards that comply with federal regulations to protect against the loss, misuse or alteration of information that we have collected from you.

## Contact Information

If you have questions about this CME activity, please contact Diane Frost at the University of Nebraska Medical Center, Center for Continuing Education by phone at 402-559-5145 or by email at dfrost@unmc.edu

## Method of Participation/How to Receive Credit

The content of this CME activity is divided into three Modules that together comprise 7.25 *AMA PRA Category 1 Credits™*.

Each Module may be taken separately for individual credit, as follows:

Module 1: "Risk Assessment, Patient Selection, and Treatment Planning"
Chapters 1 through 3 (2.25 credits)
Module 2: "Initiating, Documenting, Monitoring, and Discontinuing Opioid Therapy"
Chapter 4 through 6 (3 credits)
Module 3: "Managing Special Risk Populations and Situations"
Chapters 7 through 10 (2 credits)

While it is recommended that these Modules be taken sequentially, participants may elect to take whatever Modules best meet their educational needs.

**CME credit for this activity is free.** There is no charge to participants for earning CME credit, regardless of how many Modules they may elect to take.

In order to receive credit, participants should complete the following steps:

1. Read the chapters included in each Module.
2. Go online to www.fsmb.org/CME
3. Click on the link to: "Claim Credit for *Responsible Opioid Prescribing: A Clinician's Guide*"
4. Enter the following *case-sensitive* Access Code to enter the online post-test and to claim credit: FSMBCME
5. Select the Module you would like to access to claim credit for, and complete the online registration process. You will be asked to select your own user name and password upon registration. You will only need to register one time to complete all three Modules. Simply enter the user name and password you selected when registering upon subsequent visits.
6. Complete and submit the online post-test and evaluation form. Participants must correctly answer at least 80% of the questions in order to receive credit.
7. Your CME certificate will be issued to the screen upon successful completion. Please print your CME certificate.

# Responsible Opioid Prescribing™

## A CLINICIAN'S GUIDE

### SECOND EDITION
### REVISED AND EXPANDED

# Contents

# Illustrations

# Introduction
## *How To Use This Book*

*Responsible Opioid Prescribing: A Clinician's Guide* will help practitioners understand and implement practices that support rational, transparent, and risk-managed opioid prescribing. The recommendations in this book are grounded in two well-respected and widely adopted guidance documents. (See Appendix A and Appendix B.)

- The Federation of State Medical Boards (FSMB) "Model Policy for the Use of Controlled Substances for the Treatment of Pain."
- "Clinical Guidelines for the Use of Chronic Opioid Therapy in Chronic Noncancer Pain," a joint effort of the American Pain Society (APS) and the American Academy of Pain Medicine (AAPM).

Over the past decade, many medical specialty societies and organizations have formulated guidelines for clinicians prescribing opioids. Links to many of the most recent of these are listed in Appendix C at the back of this book.

The FSMB Model Policy is a succinct seven-point summary of recommendations about patient evaluation, treatment plans, periodic review, and other aspects of managing patients in pain. Originally formulated in 1998 and updated in 2003, FSMB's Model Policy is currently being reviewed and updated by a panel of experts in pain and addiction medicine. FSMB expects to issue a revised version of the Model Policy in 2013.

The APS-AAPM guidelines, published in 2009, resulted from the commissioning of an expert panel to review the evidence related to the use of long-term opioid therapy for chronic noncancer pain. The panel concluded that evidence of efficacy of long-term opioid therapy is limited. However, it can be an effective therapy for carefully selected and monitored patients. The panel noted that opioids are also associated with potentially serious harm, including opioid-related adverse effects and outcomes related to misuse.*

---

\* Although the terms "substance abuse" and "substance misuse" are often used interchangeably, I prefer, when possible, to use "misuse" because "abuse" has a narrower meaning than "misuse," which encompasses not only self-harming use (i.e., abuse) but also medical misuse, non-medical use, and diversion, all issues that are relevant to the topics presented in this book.

The FSMB Model Policy is intended to guide medical boards that evaluate and regulate physician practice while the APS-AAPM guidelines go into greater clinical and pharmacological depth and address important topics such as patient selection and monitoring, methadone treatment, pregnancy, psychotherapeutic co-interventions, and breakthrough pain.

The chapters of this book expand greatly on both of these documents and translate the recommendations into clear steps that can be implemented in real-world clinical practice.

Many clinicians already perform many of the key steps recommended in both the FSMB Model Policy and the APS-AAPM Guidelines. Most clinicians, for example, evaluate their patients, specify goals of therapy, document findings and prescriptions, and create treatment plans of some kind. Safe, responsible opioid prescribing doesn't mean learning an entirely new way of practicing medicine. It means learning to apply principles of good medicine to the specific challenges of opioids and the patients undergoing long-term opioid therapy. While the paradigm of chronic disease management can and should be generalized to chronic pain care, the fact that opioids have misuse potential brings an added dimension to this treatment modality, requiring an additional focus on safe use. By taking simple steps to ensure that opioids are prescribed safely and transparently, clinicians can help their patients achieve better outcomes, as well as protect themselves should they encounter the scrutiny of regulators.

Regulators and law enforcement agencies, such as the U.S. Drug Enforcement Administration (DEA), have urged prescribers to be vigilant when prescribing abusable drugs, particularly for patients with known or suspected risk of misuse. Vigilant and responsible opioid prescribing requires clinicians to become well-versed in the latest guidance on how to evaluate and select patients for whom opioids are appropriate, how to structure treatment outcomes and expectations, how to monitor patients, and how to manage the various complications that can arise when opioids are prescribed.

In November 2011, the U.S. Food and Drug Administration (FDA) released its Risk Evaluation and Mitigation Strategies (REMS) content guidelines for prescriber education.[1] At the same time, the White House Office of National Drug Control Policy, in collaboration with other branches of the federal government, introduced the "Action Plan

To Address National Prescription Drug Abuse Epidemic."[2] Like this book, their plan seeks to strike a "balance between cracking down on Drug Diversion and protecting delivery of effective pain management."

The joint press release from the White House, FDA, DEA, and the Department of Health and Human Services described their plan as providing "a national framework for reducing prescription drug diversion and misuse by supporting the expansion of state-based prescription drug monitoring programs, recommending more convenient and environmentally responsible disposal methods to remove unused medications from the home, supporting education for patients and healthcare providers, and reducing the prevalence of pill mills and doctor shopping through enforcement efforts."

This revised and expanded edition of *Responsible Opioid Prescribing: A Clinician's Guide* is in step with these important efforts, covering the educational themes emphasized by the FDA and the new federal plan to combat prescription drug misuse. This book is intended to offer every clinician a solid foundation for responsible and vigilant opioid prescribing.

As a physician who specializes in pain management, I am optimistic about the future of pain treatment. Opioids represent only a small part of the spectrum of options for mitigating pain, but they carry a substantial level of risk. The statistics on opioid-related misuse, diversion, morbidity, and mortality are unacceptable. I believe this is a problem humans created and humans can solve. Neither this book nor any single continuing medical education (CME) activity will eliminate the nonmedical use of opioids and the often-tragic consequences of that misuse. But I believe we can—and must—educate ourselves about how to improve our practices to minimize misuse and diversion, while at the same time providing the best pain management possible. We are obliged, as medical professionals, to make the clinician-patient interface an opportunity for reducing the risks associated with opioid therapy, and for increasing patient understanding of those risks.

In an era when under-treated pain and prescription drug misuse are both severe public health problems, clinicians may respond in either of two unsatisfactory ways. Some may simply avoid treating patients in chronic pain. Other clinicians may be overly enthusiastic in their embrace of opioids, either not appreciating their inherent risks or believing that if a little bit of an opioid is good, then more must be better. I'm convinced that we can find a balance between a compassionate commitment to optimal pain relief and an urgent concern for the potential harm associated with any treatment. Medicine is all about managing risk, and the safe and effective use of opioids is no different. Opioids are ancient drugs that have been both glorified and demonized for centuries. It is time we learn to safely harness their health-enhancing gifts, when indicated, while maintaining a clear-eyed recognition of their potential risks.

# Chapter 1
## *The Clinician's Dilemma: Under-Treated Pain Versus Prescription Drug Misuse*

In recent years, two compelling public health trends have become entwined like the twin serpents in the caduceus: first came increased clinical attention across all medical specialties to the under-treatment of pain, generating increased prescribing of opioid analgesics. This was followed by a shift in patterns of drug misuse from illicit to prescription drugs—most notably a dramatic rise in diversion and non-medical use of opioid pain medications within the United States.

As the gatekeepers of prescription medications, clinicians are being enlisted to fight on two fronts: combating pain, while simultaneously defending against the misuse of and addiction to opioid pain medications. Some clinicians bristle at adding "pharmacovigilance" and "risk management" to their already lengthy task list. But the combination of potential therapeutic benefit and high risk associated with opioid analgesics leaves us no alternative but to become more committed and sophisticated risk managers.

The practice of medicine is often a balancing act. Nowhere is this truer than in the treatment of patients in pain. Pain is the most common reason patients seek care, and treating pain often presents clinicians with significant challenges —not least of which is the fact that pain is always subjective. None of us can prove that someone does or does not have pain. It is always an "untestable hypothesis."

Opioids are potent and reliable pain relievers, but they are not a panacea. Opioids do not work for all pain, or for all patients, and they may cause adverse effects ranging from mild to life threatening. The primary clinical goal is to balance the legitimate need to treat the harm that comes with ongoing pain with the equally compelling need to minimize other risks of harm, to both the patient and society at large.

Over the past two decades, clinicians who treat patients in pain have been buffeted by the winds of both data and opinion, alternately pushing pain management towards and away from opioid therapy. Prior to the 1990s, clinicians often viewed opioid pain medications with skepticism and avoided prescribing them, even when risks were thought to be low. This perspective gave way to the recognition that many patients were being under-treated for their pain, leading to increased interest in the clinical value of opioids and a dramatic rise in rates of opioid prescribing for pain. In her 2008 testimony to the U.S. Senate Committee on Judiciary, National Institute for Drug Abuse (NIDA) Director Nora D. Volkow, M.D., stated: *"Prescriptions for opiates have escalated from around 40 million in 1991 to nearly 180 million in 2007, with the U.S. their biggest consumer. The U.S. has supplied 99 percent of the world total for hydrocodone (e.g., Vicodin) and 71 percent of oxycodone (e.g., OxyContin)."*[3] Today, opioids are the most-prescribed class of prescription medications in the United States, with hydrocodone as the single most prescribed drug in the US. Factors contributing to the rise in opioid prescribing include the introduction of long-acting formulations and novel delivery systems, as well as prescriber concerns over the dangers of non-opioid analgesics such as non-steroidal anti-inflammatory drugs (NSAIDS).

Escalating opioid prescribing rates coincided with a dramatic rise in diversion and nonmedical use of these powerful drugs, perhaps due in part to the misconception by abusers that prescription medications are less dangerous than illicit drugs. Another potential contributory factor was the proliferation of hundreds of rogue Internet sites where consumers could purchase opioid medications without prescriptions, or via "online consultations" with real or bogus physicians. Meanwhile, "pill mills" where opioids are prescribed indiscriminately to anyone who would pay, proliferated in states such as Florida and Kentucky. Alarming spikes in addiction and unintended overdose deaths paralleled heightened prescribing rates of opioid medications.

It remains unclear exactly how much of this problem of misuse, addiction, and unintended overdose death is related to well-intended, but possibly under-informed or under-educated prescribers who over-prescribe opioids for legitimate patients in pain.

The winds of clinical, regulatory, and public opinion are now pushing clinicians toward a more cautious approach to opioid prescribing with a greater emphasis on risk management. This paradigm shift is being driven by undeniably dire statistics that reveal the scope of devastation caused by inappropriate use of opioid medications.

Clinicians, however, still face the challenge of balancing the real need for pain control with the need to minimize and manage the risks associated with opioid analgesics. My view is that this balancing act is not so different from the decisions required when clinicians use many other potentially risky pharmacological therapies. Solid medical practice is founded upon making rational and individualized decisions based on risk-benefit analyses, and I believe we can make these medical decisions about controlled substances in a manner that best serves the interests of our patients and society at large. In the early days of general anesthesia use, anesthesia-related morbidity and mortality occurred at unacceptable rates. Many thought anesthesia was too dangerous because clinicians had not yet learned how to use this tool safely. Many indispensible drugs have high risks. But over time, the medical community has established safe parameters for their use in appropriate cases.

Employing effective risk management is simply good medicine. Clinicians routinely use dangerous treatments—such as NSAIDS, carbamazepine, chemotherapy, and even insulin, to cite just a few examples—and we do so only when the potential benefits outweigh the risks. We use great care to deliver these risky therapies safely. The challenge posed by opioid analgesics is that not only are they potentially dangerous for patients, they are highly sought-after for misuse.

Prescribing opioid analgesics responsibly should not require that clinicians stake out polarized positions on the issues. Opioids are neither inherently "good" nor inherently "bad." Nor is there any need to be "pro" or "con" when it comes to opioids. All clinicians can agree that we must support the use of opioids in those cases where it is in the patient's best interest and oppose it when it is not. Your medical judgment, founded on prudent and shared medical decision-making, must weigh the potential risks and benefits of opioid therapy against alternative treatment options. The risk of non-treatment must also be included in this risk-benefit analysis. In daily practice, that means a prescriber may be "pro" opioid for one patient and "con" for another. This book provides a practical foundation for clinicians to perform the balancing act required in opioid management for persistent pain.

## Prescription Drug Misuse

The chapters to come will describe how clinicians can implement responsible opioid prescribing in their busy daily practices. But first,

I want to be sure you fully appreciate the magnitude of the current problems with prescription drug misuse. Let's be clear: the misuse of prescription opioid drugs in the United States has created a significant and growing public health crisis of addiction, overdose, and death. The opioid medications associated with these problems include immediate and extended release products, as well as methadone. Many people directly affected by the crisis have been previously healthy and have had no history of substance misuse.[4]

If nothing you've read or heard so far has focused your mind on this public health crisis, the following statistics should:

- Between 1998 and 2008, the rate of opioid misuse increased 400%.[5]
- More than 6 million Americans are abusing prescription drugs— more than the number abusing cocaine, heroin, hallucinogens, and inhalants, combined.[6]
- Emergency-room visits related to pharmaceutical opioids doubled between 2004 and 2008.[7]
- Between 1998 and 2008, there was a fivefold increase in drug treatment admissions for prescription opioids.[8]
- The number of deaths nationwide attributable to prescription opioid analgesics quadrupled between 1999 and 2007.[7]
- From 1999 to 2005 the number of hospital records related to poisoning deaths mentioning methadone increased 468%.[9]
- Opioid overdose is now the second-leading cause of accidental death in America, exceeded only by car crashes; in 17 states opioid overdose is the leading cause of accidental death.[10]

Behind these figures lie millions of tragic stories of untimely death, fractured families, shattered dreams, and wasted lives. The same spectrum of ills can be found in the wake of any abused drug, including alcohol, tobacco, heroin, and cocaine, to name just a few. But the fact that opioids are *prescription* drugs makes it imperative that prescribers become more vigilant risk managers as they care for patients in pain.

## The Continuing Need for Pain Management

Given the magnitude of the problems related to opioid analgesics, it can be tempting to resort to draconian solutions: clinicians may simply stop prescribing opioids, or legislation intended to improve pharmacovigilance may inadvertently curtail patient access to care.

As we work to reduce diversion and misuse of prescription opioids, it's critical to remember that the problem of unrelieved pain remains as urgent as ever.

Medicine and public health measures have succeeded in greatly increasing longevity. But although we live longer as a population, we do not necessarily live better. A 2011 congressionally mandated study by the Institute of Medicine Committee on Advancing Pain Research, Care, and Education reported that *100 million Americans suffer from chronic pain*, costing up to $635 billion annually in treatment and lost productivity.[11]

Other surveys set the problem of chronic pain in stark relief:

- Among all adults 65 years of age and over who reported pain lasting more than 24 hours, 60% stated that it lasted more than one year.[11]
- In 2004, more than 25% of adults 18 years of age and over reported low back pain in the past 3 months, with high rates of limited activity and serious psychological distress.[12]
- Low back pain is the second most common neurological ailment in the US behind headache (when every type and severity level of headache are lumped together).[13]
- The incidence of pain in the US is greater than that of diabetes, heart disease and cancer *combined*.[13, 14]
- Tragically, research shows that 50-70% of patients die in moderate to severe pain, despite the availability of opioids and other therapies to control pain.[15]

Without doubt, there *have* been improvements in pain treatment in recent years. Significant efforts have begun to reduce the incidence of untreated or under-treated pain in children, older patients, and in all other vulnerable patient populations. The following general principles are now widely accepted for pain management, according to current clinical guidelines, policy statements, and organizational goals:[16]

- Pain management is integral to good medical practice for all patients.
- Opioid therapy to relieve pain and improve function is legitimate medical practice for acute and chronic pain of both cancer and non-cancer origins.
- Patients should not be denied opioid medications except when the risks outweigh the potential benefits.

- The use of opioids for other than legitimate medical purposes poses a threat to the individual and society.
- Prescribers have a responsibility to minimize the potential for the misuse and diversion of controlled substances.

Although pain remains the most common reason a patient seeks medical attention, most clinicians are grossly under-trained in pain assessment, pain management, and appropriate use of controlled substances. Four factors contribute to the ongoing problem of both under-treated pain and opioid over-prescribing:

1. Lack of knowledge among prescribers about current pain management guidelines, risk management practices, and research in pain medicine.
2. Lack of knowledge among prescribers about addiction, dependence, and misuse.
3. The perception that prescribing adequate amounts of opioids (high or low dosages) will result in unnecessary scrutiny by regulatory authorities.
4. Lack of understanding of regulatory policies and processes.

To these factors might be added a fifth: the absence of a clearly stated overview of how government regulations and professional guidelines for prescribing can be incorporated into the hectic daily practice of clinicians. This book answers this critical need.

## Responsible Prescribing With Incomplete Data

Although both the problem of prescription drug misuse and the need for adequate pain relief are evident, clear clinical data to guide practitioners in balanced and responsible opioid prescribing remain elusive. But the absence of complete information about the risks and benefits of opioids does not relieve practitioners of the obligation to treat patients as safely and effectively as possible. Practicing medicine with incomplete and sometimes conflicting data is familiar territory for primary care and specialist clinicians alike, whether treating cardiac disease, cancer, or chronic pain. We remain obliged to treat pain as best we can, given the state of research, and to become and remain as well-informed as possible about the risks and benefits of specific medications. That's what this book is all about.

Many difficult issues regarding the use of opioids remain poorly supported, one way or the other, by clear science. In the chapters to come, I'll deal with many of the challenges presented by vexing questions that have limited science in guiding clinical practice, such as the efficacy of opioids in chronic pain, rates of and concerns about addiction and misuse, and dose escalation and discontinuation.

The evidence supporting long-term efficacy for opioid use in chronic noncancer pain is limited and of low quality. The 2009 APS-AAPM Clinical Guidelines For the Use of Chronic Opioid Therapy in Chronic Noncancer Pain concluded that clinical data on efficacy are currently not adequate to support or refute the role this treatment should play for any given individual (Appendix B). In addition, the rate of addiction or misuse in patients given opioids for chronic pain is commonly questioned. It was previously believed that addiction associated with opioids for chronic pain was rare. The data upon which these conclusions were drawn, however, have been found to be inadequate and seriously flawed. Although we currently do not know the exact rate of addiction in patients legitimately prescribed opioids for pain or the rate of overall misuse, we know that rates are high enough that they should be considered a significant potential adverse effect.

Addiction and misuse are often a major concern associated with opioid use. Opioids, however, have a wide range of potential adverse effects that can predispose a patient to serious morbidity and mortality. Much of this risk relates to respiratory depression, potentially leading to unintended overdose, negative impact on endocrine function, and possibly, heightened fracture risk related to effects on bone metabolism and from falls. Risk is increased among the elderly; those with impaired renal or hepatic function; individuals with cardiopulmonary disorders, such as chronic obstructive pulmonary disease (COPD); congestive heart failure (CHF), sleep apnea, or mental illness; and in patients who combine opioids with other respiratory depressants such as alcohol, sedative-hypnotics, benzodiazepines, or barbiturates.

In cases where patients do not respond to long-term opioid therapy, some clinicians routinely escalate the dose, hoping that higher doses will either achieve the desired analgesia or overcome pharmacological tolerance. Many clinicians were taught that there was no ceiling dose with opioids, and to titrate up until pain was relieved (or there were intolerable side effects). Escalating dosages as a reflexive response to poor efficacy, however, is a serious mistake. Patients who do not respond to a trial of opioids, with structured dose titration and monitoring, must be evaluated to determine whether or not the pain is responsive to opioids, whether efficacy is limited because of side effects or inadequate dosing, or whether misuse or diversion is possible. Scientific data are inadequate to guide us in one direction or another but common sense can help to a great extent. We know that dose escalation comes with increased risk, so when increased dosing is thought to be warranted, we must proportionately raise our vigilance, with a clear view toward indicators of efficacy in the absence of indicators of adverse effects or aberrant use. Prescribers must develop distinct, measurable end-points for their treatment plans (e.g., functional capacities, exercise tolerance, sleep, mood, social interaction), and they must be as willing to *discontinue* therapy as they are to initiate it. A structured approach to discontinuing opioid therapy (commonly referred to as an "exit strategy") should be part of treatment planning at dose initiation.

Starting opioid therapy can be easier than stopping it. But, if you are not prepared to stop the treatment—if it does not work, if the chronic pain syndrome subsides, or if its risk outweighs its benefits—you probably should not start it. Discontinuing a long-term opioid regime is easiest at the earliest signs of ineffectiveness, intolerance, or aberrant use. Assessment of efficacy and safety should occur before dosages rise to high levels, as high dosages require clear evidence of benefit without adverse outcomes or aberrant patient behavior. Long-term opioid therapy that continues without clear evidence of benefit, or despite evidence of adversity or aberrant use, may contribute to an iatrogenic problem where tapering becomes more difficult, or requires protracted periods of time or specialized intervention.

In an effort to guide healthcare providers in the context of unanswered research questions, the Centers for Disease Control and Prevention (CDC) in 2010 issued the following recommendations, which it acknowledged are based on promising interventions and expert opinion, not rigorous evidence-based research:[10]

- Use opioid medications for acute or chronic pain only after determining that alternative therapies do not deliver adequate pain relief. The lowest effective dose of opioids should be used.
- In addition to behavioral screening and use of patient contracts, consider random, periodic, urine testing for opioids and other drugs

for any patient less than 65 years old with noncancer pain who is being treated with opioids for more than six weeks.

- If a patient's dosage has increased to ≥120 morphine milligram equivalents per day without substantial improvement in pain and function, seek a consult from a pain specialist.
- Do not prescribe long-acting or controlled-release opioids (e.g., OxyContin®, fentanyl patches, and methadone) for acute pain.
- Periodically request a report from your state prescription drug monitoring program on the prescribing of opioids to your patients by other providers.

All of these points will be explored in more depth in later chapters. For now, let me briefly summarize the fundamental tenets of responsible opioid prescribing, as presented in this book, which expand upon the CDC recommendations:

## Summary
### PATIENT EVALUATION AND SELECTION
- Reserve long-term opioid therapy for patients who have tried other potentially effective treatments that pose less risk, including physical therapy, exercise, cognitive-behavioral therapy, and non-opioid analgesics.
- Screen patients before and during treatment for risks of all adverse outcomes, including those with mental illness and substance misuse, cardiopulmonary disease, and endocrine disorders.
- Understand that patients may be reluctant to disclose a history of substance misuse. Always check the medical record, a prescription drug-monitoring database, and third parties within the allowable circle of care.
- Don't start long-term use of opioids by default. Long-term opioid prescribing should generally be reserved for persistent or chronic pain and should only occur after careful patient selection, discussion of risks, and the setting of realistic expectations and functional goals.
- Educate patients about the risks and benefits of opioid medications, as well as about their proper storage and disposal, so that they can make informed decisions about choosing or rejecting opioid therapy.

**TREATMENT PLANS**

- Be sure that the decision to start treatment is clearly agreed to by the patient and prescriber, and that each is informed about (and is willing to work toward) treatment continuation or discontinuation, based on functional goals and safety.

- Explain to patients that opioids used to treat acute pain are for time-limited use. At the outset, set expectations that opioids should be discontinued when the pain problem is no longer acute.

- Avoid dispensing more medication than necessary. A 30-day supply for acute pain may be more than necessary. In treating acute pain with opioids, give only the amount believed to be needed. Be aware that excess medication may serve to stock an uncontrolled medicine cabinet and increase the risks of accidental toxicity or diversion.

- Be sure that patients understand the exit strategy if treatment needs to be discontinued.

**PERIODIC REVIEW AND MONITORING**

- Never continue long-term opioid therapy with patients who, after reasonable efforts, show inadequate progress toward functional goals.

- Consult with more specialized healthcare providers if a patient's problems exceed your range of expertise. Do not accept unmanageable risk just because the appropriate consultant may not be available.

- Don't abandon patients with aberrant behaviors or a prescription drug problem. Consider all possible causes for the behavior and remain open to employing other potentially safe treatments.

- Question how your patient is using his or her opioids. Some patients may not use the drugs you prescribe as directed. They may vary the dosing or combine them with other dangerous substances, drugs, or alcohol in ways that are not advisable.

- Have clear treatment parameters beyond which continued use requires re-evaluation. For instance, acute pain that continues to require opioid therapy should be fully re-evaluated.

- Exercise compassion and trust—but verify. Recognize that misuse and addiction often coincide with denial and a striking lack of insight. Clinicians, therefore, must use all available tools to discern these problems as early as possible. This includes closely monitoring functional and behavioral status, utilizing urine toxicity screens and prescription drug monitoring systems, and remaining engaged in care before and after any potential adverse outcomes.

In the rest of this book I will "unpack" these bullet points with an eye to the real-world, day-to-day demands made on clinicians like you and me. Although the challenges of balancing the potential benefits and risks of opioids are real, they're no different than the choices presented by potentially risky treatments in other spheres of medical practice. As you will see, responsible opioid prescribing often relies on subtle changes of attitude, relatively simple changes to policies or procedures, and a willingness to examine one's current approach to opioids. When opioids are prescribed responsibly, both patients and clinicians benefit.

# Chapter 2
## *Effective Patient Evaluation: Assessment and Selection*

A t the core of the requirement to evaluate patients thoroughly is a paradox: although a clinician can take a history, do a physical examination, consider past treatments, probe for a history of substance misuse, and note coexisting diseases, he or she cannot measure or even objectively confirm the pain that a patient is experiencing. Despite modern diagnostic and evaluative tools, such as magnetic resonance imaging (MRI), ultrasonography, and electromyography, pain remains an untestable hypothesis. Perhaps one reason that prescribers are reluctant to aggressively treat pain has to do with the often-frustrating fact that we can't prove that someone is or is not in pain, just as we can't prove the presence or absence of pain relief. As Elaine Scarry notes in her book *The Body in Pain*:[17] "To hear about pain is to have doubt; to experience pain is to have certainty." In the end, treaters must accept the maxim "Pain is what a patient says it is." Anyone complaining of pain is suffering from something; the clinician's job is to try to figure out the cause of the suffering and to formulate a plan for reversing its erosion of the patient's quality of life. However, it must be said that there are some patients who present with reports of pain who are neither legitimate patients nor intend to use opioids for legitimate medical purposes.

Today it is widely recognized that pain is never simply "physical" or "psychological." The mind is always involved in a patient's experience of pain, and it can magnify or diminish pain perception. The almost complete overlap between the medication groups used by psychiatrists and pain specialists attests to the inextricable links between mind and body that make meaningless the cliché phrase "the pain is all in your head." Figure 1 shows that there is no psychopharmacological drug group that is not also known to have some analgesic effects—even if each drug group is not an ideal choice for treating pain.

**FIGURE 1. OVERLAPPING ANALGESIC AND PSYCHIATRIC DRUG GROUPS**

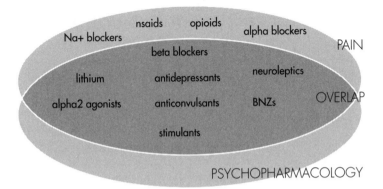

## Assessing Pain

Pain measurement scales, such as the familiar 0 to 10 numerical pain scale (Figure 2) or the "faces" pain rating scale (Figure 3) provide some guidance about a patient's experience of pain intensity, but all are open to wide variations among individuals and within an individual at different times.

Multidimensional instruments, such as the McGill Pain Questionnaire or the Brief Pain Inventory, provide a broader picture of a patient's experience than the pain scales just mentioned. (See Appendix D.) Several of these instruments are available on the FSMB website in the Resource section: http://www.fsmb.org/pain-resources.html. But pain assessment tools may be cumbersome to administer in a busy clinic setting, and in the end, suffer the same limitations as all other attempts to measure pain. If either the number scales or face scales become difficult for patients, I like to fall back on asking them to use simple descriptors such as mild, moderate, or severe to describe their pain. Although any of these reports are intrinsically subjective, it may be extremely valuable to use these values or descriptions to evaluate the impact of any given intervention.

The basic pain assessment includes core elements, most of which are traditional features of a patient workup. These include chief complaint; history of present illness; past medical, surgical, and psychosocial history; family history; physical examination; and examination of imaging and other diagnostic studies or tests. Tailoring this

**FIGURE 2: STANDARD VISUAL ANALOG SCALE (VAS) FOR PAIN**

| 1 | 2 | 3 | 4 | 5 | 6 | 7 | 8 | 9 | 10 |
|---|---|---|---|---|---|---|---|---|---|
| NO PAIN | | | | MODERATE PAIN | | | | | WORST PAIN POSSIBLE |

Adapted From: Goodwin J, Bajwa ZH. Evaluating the patient with chronic pain. In: *Principles and Practice of Pain Medicine 2nd Ed.* Warfield CA, and Bajwa ZH., Eds. 2004. New York, NY, McGraw-Hill Companies, Inc. Page 65, column 1, paragraph 3.

**FIGURE 3: FACES SCALE FOR PAIN**

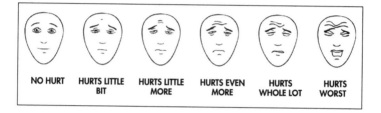

| NO HURT | HURTS LITTLE BIT | HURTS LITTLE MORE | HURTS EVEN MORE | HURTS WHOLE LOT | HURTS WORST |

Source: *PAIN 2001*; 93:173-183. Used with permission from International Association for the Study of Pain (IASP*). The instructions for administration are currently available in more than 24 languages from www.painsourcebook.ca.

assessment to the patient in pain will mean additional focus on the pain history, including functional impact; prior analgesic approaches, therapies, or interventions; examination of those with mental illness, including tobacco, alcohol, and other substances of misuse; risk assessment; and review of relevant records, including the prescription drug monitoring system.

The best way to begin assessing a patient's pain is to ask about it and listen. This may sound trivial, but, in the hurly-burly of daily clinical life, it can be challenging. All too often clinicians become overly focused on quantifying, categorizing, and deciding how best to treat pain as a single symptom. In the process, they may not ask questions that relate to their patients' global experiences of suffering. In doing so, they may unintentionally distance themselves from their patients. By focusing narrowly on a disease or symptom, they can lose the "big picture" of the whole person and thus miss important diagnostic clues that could lead to more effective interventions.

---

**SETTING UP YOUR PAIN MANAGEMENT PRACTICE**

Prescribing controlled substances such as opioids requires compliance with relevant laws and regulations. Learning about these requirements and arranging your practice to accommodate them will make the entire pain management process go more smoothly. Here are some suggestions:

- Contact your state medical board for guidance on state regulations related to prescribing controlled substances.
- Understand your state's prescription monitoring program.
- Review the Federal Controlled Substances Act.
- Conduct in-house training for all staff about legal and regulatory issues related to controlled substances.

---

Three relatively simple steps can **vastly** improve taking a history from a patient in pain:

1. Take control of time;
2. Focus on the patient, not the pain; and
3. Use reflective listening skills.

These steps can help connect the clinician with the patient, as well as improve patient selectivity, evaluation, and the efficacy of any chosen analgesic treatments.

### STEP 1: TAKE CONTROL OF TIME

Clinicians are increasingly pressured to see more and more patients. This "time crunch" often becomes apparent with patients in pain. Such patients typically have complex presentations and histories. Nonetheless, clinicians must relentlessly look under every "rock" for clues, and withhold judgment until ample evidence is acquired. This unavoidably time-consuming process can cause practitioners to perceive pain patients as "difficult."

Unfortunately, these challenges can lead clinicians in exactly the wrong direction. Instead of allotting increased time and patience to the diagnostic task, prescribers confronted with "difficult" patients may speed up, and either consciously or unconsciously, rush to judgment in an effort to minimize time spent with an emotionally sensitive, demanding, or frustrated patient. Effective patient selection and evaluation, in other words, requires a commitment to spending enough time and attention to what the patient is saying both verbally and through non-verbal behaviors.

### STEP 2: FOCUS ON THE PATIENT, NOT THE PAIN

In taking a history about pain, clinicians should ask questions not only about the pain itself (e.g., its location, intensity, duration), but also about the pain's collateral impact on the patient's life. To use a musical metaphor, you need to listen not just to the lyrics (the self-evident parts of what the patient says), but to the music as well (the less obvious verbal and nonverbal messages about their feelings, fears, expectations, goals, etc.). Clinicians need to be alert to subtle warning signs of trouble and take the time to ask follow-up questions.

Pain is usually interwoven with unpleasant experiences such as fatigue, nausea, depression, and anxiety. Recognizing these elements of the pain cycle is vital for understanding the true dimensions of a patient's experience and for choosing the most effective means of alleviating his or her suffering. For example, depression can dramatically alter pain perception—almost always for the worse. Patients may not offer unprompted information about their depression out of fear that the clinician will think their pain is "all in their head." If you don't ask direct questions related to mood, or pick up on the subtle signs from the patient's answers that suggest psychosocial deterioration, you may not recognize this significant factor in the experience of pain. Similarly, many other aspects of a person's life can affect his or her pain, such as the use or misuse of licit or illicit drugs, high stress levels at work or home, or physical deconditioning because of a lack of activity.

### STEP 3: USE REFLECTIVE LISTENING SKILLS

Pain undermines one's ability to cope with the ups and downs of normal life, and patients in pain are frequently more emotional than they might be otherwise. Pain can make anybody defensive, short-tempered, or even hostile. In addition, by the time they see a clinician, pain patients may have undergone previous treatments that either were ineffective or that actually made things worse. In some cases, the tension may be palpable, and in others, it may simply be suppressed. In all cases, though, the patient in pain wants and needs to be believed and validated. In a sense, treatment actually begins during the process of evaluation and selection.

An effective strategy for collecting a comprehensive history and building a successful patient-clinician relationship is *reflective listening*. This means listening carefully and non-judgmentally to what your patient is saying, then reflecting it back in a slightly modified or reframed manner. This allows the clinician to confirm the accuracy of his or her beliefs. It also assures patients that they are being heard and gives them a chance to correct mistaken beliefs or perceptions that could affect their care.

Using a reflective listening strategy may be easier said than done. If a patient says something at odds with the evidence, or uses threatening or hostile language, one's natural reaction is to immediately defend oneself, rebut the charges, or deny the underlying assumptions. This can quickly create confrontation or a power struggle that can be difficult to overcome. It is much more effective to take a moment before responding, and then to consciously try to simply restate what the patient just said.

For example, a patient may angrily say "Doctor, those pills you gave me don't work—I told you before that I need something stronger." Even in cases where you suspect the patient may be angling for stronger and possibly riskier medications for spurious reasons, a directly confrontational response may backfire. It may be best to say something like: "You seem to be irritated with me because you don't think the medications I prescribed are working for you. Let's see if we can get to the bottom of this." Reflective listening responses such as this provide several advantages:

- They are less likely to evoke or exacerbate patient defensiveness.
- They encourage the patient to keep talking to reveal more about his or her true motives.
- They communicate respect, caring, and compassion, and encourage a therapeutic alliance.
- They open an opportunity for the patient to correct misunderstandings or clarify exactly what he or she means.

Although reflective listening can be particularly helpful when a patient is emotional, it is a useful approach for following up on or probing answers to questions that you ask during any patient encounter.

# Elements of a Comprehensive History

Comprehensive evaluation of a patient in pain usually requires moving beyond the typical list of questions asked during a general history. It may be possible to gather this information well before an in-person visit. Standardized questionnaires can efficiently capture much-needed information as long as the clinician is prepared in advance for the patient in pain. In most cases where pain is the chief complaint, it is certainly appropriate to begin a conversation by asking about the pain, but then it is usually best to review the broader context and impact of that pain. Here are some points that may be useful to cover in an initial evaluation:

- Location of pain
- Character of pain (i.e., shooting or stinging, continuous or intermittent, worse at night or in the morning)
- Lowest and highest pain on 0 to 10 scale in a typical day
- Usual pain on 0 to 10 scale on a typical day (augmented by verbal descriptors)
- How and when pain started
- Exacerbating and relieving factors (i.e., stress, alcohol, other medical concerns)
- Effect of pain on sleep
- Effect of pain on mood
- Effect of pain on functioning at work
- Effect of pain on quality of personal life, such as relationships, sex, or recreation
- Is the patient involved in a legal or protracted insurance process connected to his or her chronic pain, such as a motor vehicle accident or a disability case?
- What activities could the patient do before pain impacted his or her life that he or she can't do now?
- What does the patient expect from medications or other treatments in terms of analgesia or recovered function?
- Review of past experience/exposure to opioids
- Review of past medical/surgical history
- Review of family medical history
- Assessment of patient history of drug, alcohol, and tobacco use
- Psychosocial evaluation (including history of mental illness)

In the course of your conversations with patients, be alert to signs that they are minimizing their pain. Although it may seem counterintuitive, some patients fail to convey the true nature and severity of their pain, which can undermine the effectiveness of their treatment. They may not want to disappoint their treating clinician or offer a distraction from curing their primary disease. Some may think they should just "suck it up" and endure their pain, they may think pain is an inevitable part of their illness, or they may want to avoid acknowledging that their disease is progressing. Some may worry that if they mention their pain, their doctor will see them as complainers or even as drug-seekers or addicts. Many people also under-report pain because they fear that pain medications will dull their cognitive abilities, lead to addiction, or result in unmanageable side effects. Finally, some patients may believe that there is value in suffering, or that in some way they deserve to be in pain to expiate some form of "wrong-doing" or "sinfulness."

If you suspect a patient is minimizing his or her pain, reflective listening can help the patient see what you see and allow you to probe for the reasons underlying the minimizing. At some point, you might scratch your head and say something like "I wonder if you are the silent sufferer type?" Very few people are offended by being described as "stoic." It is often considered something of a compliment! Being seen as someone who is doing his or her part to bear the suffering is usually consoling. Regardless of the reasons for minimizing, using reflective listening skills can help you take a history by allowing patients to feel that they will not be judged negatively and can speak freely and candidly about their pain.

## Physical Examination

Medicare and other institutions have defined what constitutes a physical examination for purposes of coding and reimbursement, but for the purposes of patients in chronic pain who may be candidates for treatment with opioids, the FDA has recommended that providers "Complete a comprehensive history and physical examination, including assessment of psychosocial factors and family history of substance misuse, as well as special considerations for the elderly, women, children, and cultural/ethnic groups." Regulators expect to see at least a basic physical examination as part of the evaluation that leads to treatment with controlled substances. The exact components of the examination, however, are left to the medical judgment of the clinician, who is expected to have performed an examination proportionate to the diagnosis that justifies a treatment.

For instance, it might be expected that a patient treated with opioids for chronic low back pain will have at least received a basic examination of the lumbar spine and any other areas that could conceivably contribute to the symptoms. Such an examination might reveal pathology that could be amenable to other treatments—treatments that might pose less risks than opioid medications. The bottom line is that unless due diligence is evident with a documented physical examination, a prescriber's decision to begin a treatment that carries risk may be questioned.

Part of any physical examination involving a complaint of pain is an assessment of the patient's nervous system with focus on sensory function. Clinicians should assess for allodynia (pain from stimulation that would not normally evoke pain, such as light touch), hyperalgesia (amplified pain response to stimulation that would normally evoke only mild pain, such as gentle contact with the tip of a pin), or pain insensitivity. A sensory examination could include response to light touch, light pressure, pinprick, cold or vibration.

## Psychosocial Evaluation

Pain affects every aspect of a patient's life. It's vital, therefore, to include as part of any assessment an evaluation of the ways pain may be impacting or may be affected by psychosocial elements of a patient's life. You must be alert for signs of depression or anxiety, which are very common. Be particularly alert for suicidal thoughts since the risk of suicide is roughly double for patients with chronic pain.[18] A patient with active suicidal thoughts requires rapid assessment by a qualified professional. Standardized instruments for gathering a psychiatric history are widely available. Referral to a mental-health professional is warranted if your judgment suggests the patient has active psychological issues beyond your expertise.

Clinicians should also ask questions that will elicit information about how the patient's family system is being affected by the pain he or she is experiencing. Family or relationship dynamics can be severely eroded by the work and stress involved with supporting or coping with a person in chronic pain. Finally, clinicians should assess the ways a chronic pain condition affects the patient's work and social activities. If a pain condition is related to (or is perceived as being related to) a work-related injury, the patient may be dealing with many layers of emotional, legal, or administrative challenges. Evaluating these challenges and addressing them during treatment (for instance by referral to a vocational counselor or social worker) is just as important as treating the more direct medical issues that might be part of a painful condition.

## Evaluating Patients for the Possibility of Addiction, Diversion, or Drug Misuse

All patients complaining of pain are suffering from something and deserve a clinician's empathy and compassion. But a small minority of people seeking treatment may not actually be suffering from pain. Instead, they may be using drugs to cope with other aspects of their lives or they may be suffering from addiction or some other kind of psychological dysfunction. Although such patients may evoke strong negative reactions from clinicians, they are not "bad" people. Focusing on the patient as the problem may not help you move forward. Instead, frame the issue in terms of risks versus benefits, where the treatment being sought (i.e., opioids) is unlikely to remedy the real problem the patient has (i.e., addiction). Indeed, the "treatment" in some cases, such as addiction, is likely to do much more harm than good.

Evaluating patients for their risk of addiction or drug misuse is an essential component of any pain evaluation and requires constant vigilance without impulsively rushing to judgment. This is not unusual for clinicians. For instance, there is an old adage that if you don't suspect a pulmonary embolism, you'll never catch one. The same level of suspicion (without judgment) applies to the assessment of the patient in pain. If you don't suspect the possibility that someone who asks for an opioid might have a problem with drug misuse, you may miss a valuable opportunity to help the patient. The situation is analogous to having a patient who asks for help with excessive thirst and urination and not considering the possibility that the patient has diabetes.

Although it may sound contradictory to exhort clinicians to be empathic and supportive while simultaneously strongly probing for the truth (including information that the patient may not want to reveal), this is not such a difficult balance to achieve in daily practice. You can maintain a tolerant, nonjudgmental, and concerned posture yet remain persistent in your quest for the valid information required for prudent decision-making.

Whenever a clinician considers treating pain with a controlled substance, such as an opioid, risk of misuse or diversion is always a possibility, no matter how remote, and must be assessed. Exactly who to suspect and when to be proactive in investigating risk factors is an area of great debate. To date, no convincing data exist to support the strategy of focusing on any one specific population or setting—which means that prescribers must be vigilant with all patients. The term "universal precautions" has been applied to this approach, and in pain care, means that any patient in pain could have a drug misuse problem—just as any patient requiring a blood draw for a simple lab test could have the human immunodeficiency virus (HIV). Gourlay and Heit (2006) effectively argued that "Since there is no one behavior that is [diagnostic] of a substance use disorder, and since the prevalence of addiction in the general population is not insignificant, it is prudent to thoroughly inquire into substance use in all patients, not only those who are being treated with the opioid class of drugs. Failure to do so may leave a potentially treatable condition, such as addiction, undiagnosed and untreated."[19]

Treating everyone with the same screens, diagnostic tests, and administrative procedures can help remove bias and level the playing field so everyone is treated equally and screened thoroughly. Unfortunately,

> *What must be avoided is a rush to judgment in the absence of clear data to support such a judgment. Thus, we must often be suspicious, but rarely judgmental.*

it may be perceived by some patients and clinicians as undermining the patient-clinician relationship. Despite defensible efforts to be as consistent as possible to all, as well as to cast the broadest possible surveillance, some patients (or clinicians) may see the universal precautions approach as a sign of distrust or evidence that the patient is being presumed guilty until proven innocent. Dealing with this may require candid and clear education for patients as to why such procedures and practices are necessary and in their best interest. After all, one of a clinician's primary jobs is to be suspicious and questioning—it is part of the diagnostic quest. What must be avoided is a rush to judgment in the absence of clear data to support such judgments. Thus, we must often be suspicious, but rarely judgmental.

The presence of co-occurring pain and addiction does not preclude chronic pain management, but it does complicate it—especially if opioids are to be prescribed. It must be stressed that in these situations, most clinicians do not have the resources necessary to keep patients safe.

In evaluating pain patients for risk of addiction or signs that they may be abusing a controlled substance, it may be helpful to consider the sets of characteristics listed in Tables 1 and 2.

It's important to remember that the vast majority of patients are neither addicted nor diverting. Nonetheless, clinicians must remain vigilant for the possibility that a patient may have a problem with a controlled substance, including addiction, diversion, or any other form of misuse. Below is a list of traits that may be seen in some patients who misuse opioids. Remember that none of these behaviors alone is diagnostic, and in fact, some may be normal for a given individual.[20, 21]

- Deteriorating personal appearance and hygiene
- Appears intoxicated
- Appears sedated or confused (e.g., slurred speech, unresponsive)
- Expresses worries about addiction
- Exhibits lack of interest in rehabilitation or self-management
- Misuses alcohol or uses illicit drugs
- Arrested by police
- Victim of abuse
- Increasingly negative moods

**TABLE 1. CHARACTERISTICS OF CHRONIC-PAIN PATIENTS VERSUS ADDICTED PATIENTS**

| Chronic Pain Patient Without Addiction | Addicted Patient |
|---|---|
| Medication use is not out of control | Medication use is out of control |
| Medication use improves quality of life | Medication use impairs quality of life |
| Wants to decrease medication if adverse effects develop | Medication use continues or increases despite adverse effects |
| Is concerned about the physical problem being treated with the drug | Unaware of or in denial about any problems that develop as a result of drug treatment |
| Follows the agreement for use of the opioid | Does not follow opioid agreement |
| Frequently has left over medication | Does not have leftover medication |
| | Loses prescriptions |
| | Always has a story about why more drug is needed |

Adapted from: Webster LR, Dove B. Avoiding Opioid Abuse While Managing Pain. Sunrise River Press, North Branch, MN. 2007.

- Mood swings appear to occur at similar times of the day
- Overly reactive to admonishments or compliments
- Increasingly complains about co-workers, family, or friends
- Worsened relationships with family
- Family or significant others express concern over patient's use of analgesics
- Deliberately avoids co-workers and supervisors, especially those who have been trained to spot abusers
- Careless, makes frequent mistakes, and shows poor judgment
- Involvement in car or other accidents
- Frequent and recurring financial problems

**TABLE 2. BEHAVIORAL INDICATIONS OF ADDICTION AND PSEUDO-ADDICTION**

| (Behaviors LESS indicative of addiction) | (Behaviors MORE indicative of addiction) |
| --- | --- |
| 1. Express anxiety or desperation over recurrent symptoms | 1. Bought pain medications from a street dealer |
| 2. Hoard medications | 2. Stole money to obtain drugs |
| 3. Taken someone else's pain medications | 3. Tried to get opioids from more than one source |
| 4. Aggressively complained to doctor for more drugs | 4. Performed sex for drugs |
| 5. Requested a specific drug or medication | 5. Seen two doctors at once without them knowing |
| 6. Used more opioids than recommended | 6. Performed sex for money to buy drugs |
| 7. Drink more alcohol when in pain | 7. Stole drugs from others |
| 8. Express worry over changing to a new drug even if it offers potentially fewer side effects | 8. Prostituted others for money to obtain drugs |
| 9. Expressed concern to physician or family members that pain might lead to use of street drugs | 9. Prostituted others for drugs |
| 10. Asked for second opinion about pain medications | 10. Prescription forgery |
| 11. Smoke cigarettes to relieve pain | 11. Sold prescription drugs |
| 12. Ever used opioids to treat other symptoms | |

Adapted from: Passik SD, Kirsh KL, Donaghy KB, Portenoy R. Pain and Aberrant Drug-Related Behaviors in Medically Ill Patients With and Without Histories of Substance Abuse. *Clinical Journal of Pain* 2006;22:173–181

## Prescription Drug Monitoring Programs

In response to the problems of drug diversion and misuse of prescription medications, the federal government and many states have created prescription drug monitoring programs (PDMPs). In April 2011, President Obama announced his action plan to combat prescription drug misuse. A pillar of this plan is to expand the use of PDMPs and integrate them more fully into clinical practice. Typically, clinicians using PDMPs collect prescribing and dispensing data from pharmacies, conduct reviews and analyses of the data, and disseminate these data to appropriate regulatory and law enforcement agencies. Increasingly, these data are being made available to clinicians at the point of care with computer systems securely accessible through the Internet. (See Figure 4.)

Currently there is little uniformity, information-sharing, or cooperation among states that employ PDMPs, but efforts are under way to improve this situation. An advisory committee of the Council of State Governments has endorsed the formation of an interstate PDMP compact, and legislation to accomplish this goal is currently being drafted. If it is available to you, a PDMP may provide extremely valuable information that can help you assess a patient's status and prescription drug

**FIGURE 4. STATUS OF PRESCRIPTION DRUG MONITORING PROGRAMS (PDMPS)**

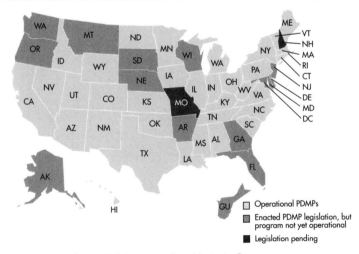

Source: Alliance of States With Prescription Drug Monitoring Programs.
Available at http://www.pmpalliance.org. Accessed January 18, 2012.

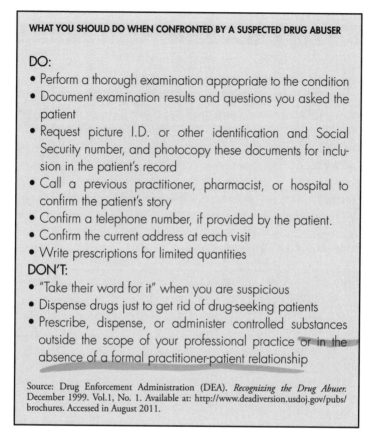

**WHAT YOU SHOULD DO WHEN CONFRONTED BY A SUSPECTED DRUG ABUSER**

**DO:**

- Perform a thorough examination appropriate to the condition
- Document examination results and questions you asked the patient
- Request picture I.D. or other identification and Social Security number, and photocopy these documents for inclusion in the patient's record
- Call a previous practitioner, pharmacist, or hospital to confirm the patient's story
- Confirm a telephone number, if provided by the patient.
- Confirm the current address at each visit
- Write prescriptions for limited quantities

**DON'T:**

- "Take their word for it" when you are suspicious
- Dispense drugs just to get rid of drug-seeking patients
- Prescribe, dispense, or administer controlled substances outside the scope of your professional practice or in the absence of a formal practitioner-patient relationship

Source: Drug Enforcement Administration (DEA). *Recognizing the Drug Abuser.* December 1999. Vol.1, No. 1. Available at: http://www.deadiversion.usdoj.gov/pubs/brochures. Accessed in August 2011.

use. By checking PDMP data (particularly for high-risk patients) clinicians can get a sense of the controlled substances that the patient has been receiving from other prescribers and other pharmacies.[22, 23]

Many tools have been developed for the formal assessment of a patient's risk of having a substance misuse problem, some of which are appropriate for routine clinical use because they are relatively brief and easily implemented. (See Table 3.) It's important to remember that currently available assessment tools are designed to identify patients who already have problems with substances, rather than predicting who might misuse drugs in the future.

**TABLE 3. TOOLS FOR PATIENT RISK ASSESSMENT**

| Tool | Use | Who Administers? | Length |
|---|---|---|---|
| Alcohol, Smoking, and Substance Involvement Screening Test (ASSIST) | Screen for current/past substance misuse | Clinician | 8 items |
| CAGE Adapted to include Drugs | Screen for current/past substance misuse | Clinician | 4 yes/no questions |
| Current Opioid Misuse Measure (COMM) | Monitor for misuse by patients currently on long-term opioid therapy | Patient self-report | 17 items |
| Diagnosis, Intractability, Risk, Efficacy (DIRE) | Screen for risk of opioid addiction | Clinician | 7 items |
| Opioid Risk Tool (ORT) | Screen for risk of opioid addiction | Clinician or patient self-report | 5 yes/no questions |
| Prescription Drug Use Questionnaire (PDUQ) | Screen for risk of opioid addiction | Clinician | 42 items |
| Pain Medication Questionnaire (PMQ) | Screen for risk of opioid addiction | Patient self-report | 26 items |
| Screening Instrument for Substance Abuse Potential (SISAP) | Screen for risk of opioid addiction/substance misuse | Clinician | 5 items |
| Screening Tool for Addiction Risk (STAR) | Screen for risk of opioid addiction/substance misuse | Patient self-report | 14 yes/no questions |
| Screener and Opioid Assessment for Patients with Pain-Revised (SOAPP-R) | Screen for risk of opioid addiction | Patient self-report | 24 items |
| Severity of Opiate Dependence Questionnaire (SODQ) | Screen for risk of opioid addiction | Patient self-report | 21 items |
| Structured Clinical Interview For Diagnostic and Statistical Manual of Mental (DSM) Disorders (SCID) | Screen for major mental disorders | Clinician | 1–2 hour assessment |

One commonly-used screening tool is called "CAGE." This classic screen was developed for alcohol misuse, but can be easily modified for any abusable drug. The questionnaire (which can be incorporated into a self-administered written assessment form) asks whether a patient has ever:

**C:** Wanted or needed to **C**ut down on drinking or drug use?

**A:** Been **A**nnoyed or **A**ngered by others complaining about the patient's drinking or drug use?

**G:** Felt **G**uilty about the consequences of the patient's drinking or drug use?

**E:** Taken a drink in the morning as an "**E**ye opener" to decrease hang-over or withdrawal?

A single positive response should elicit a clinician's caution in pre-scribing opioids to the patient. It does *not* mean opioids are completely contraindicated, just that you should raise your level of vigilance about whether or not prescribing an abusable drug is in the patient's best interest. If you deem that prescribing a controlled substance *is* appro-priate, you must exercise particular care in your informed consent, provider/patient agreement (whether verbal or written) and your risk management plan for monitoring and follow-up.

To date, no single tool has been widely endorsed or thoroughly vali-dated, and the astute clinician will recognize that the signs of misuse or addiction may not be immediately apparent in the typical clinical set-ting. If suspicion is raised for a given patient, information about previ-ous problems with substance misuse may be obtained from a collateral source, such as a family member, friend, or other healthcare professional. A clinician is not required to commence treatment until he or she is comfortable with the integrity of the situation. Understanding the signs and symptoms of misuse or addiction will help guide treatment deci-sions. In these matters it's important to respect your instincts by moving cautiously or by collecting more data when the situation warrants. Feel-ing unduly rushed by a patient into a prescribing decision may reflect a clinical problem that is worthy of review and discussion with the patient.

A complimentary approach to assessment of a patient's risk of mis-use or addiction is risk stratification. Typically, this involves assigning a patient to different levels of risk based on certain criteria. Webster et al., have suggested one such risk stratification model, illustrated in Table 4.

**TABLE 4. MATCH MONITORING TO THE PATIENT'S RISK OF DRUG ABUSE**

| Low Risk (Routine) | Moderate Risk | High Risk |
|---|---|---|
| • Pain assessment | • Biweekly visits | • Weekly visits |
| • Substance-abuse assessment | • Biweekly prescriptions | • Weekly prescriptions (on attendance) |
| • Informed consent | • Regular prescription database check | • Quarterly prescription database check |
| • Signed treatment agreement | • Third-party verification | • Third-party administration |
| • Regular follow-up visits and prescriptions | • Random urine drug screening | • Urine drug screening, scheduled and random |
| • Initial prescription database check | • Consider comorbid disease | • Consider blood screenings |
| • Medical reports | • Consider psychiatric/addiction/pain evaluation | • Psychiatric/addiction evaluation required |
| • Initial urine drug screening | • Consider medication counts | • Consider pain specialist evaluation |
| • No consultation required | • Consider limiting rapid-onset analgesics | • Limit rapid-onset analgesics |
| • Document patient-provider interactions | | • Consider limiting short-acting agents |

Source: Webster LR, Dove B. Avoiding Opioid Abuse While Managing Pain. Alliance of States With Prescription Drug Monitoring Program: Sunrise River Press. 2007.

## Assessing Risk and Benefit

Clinicians must routinely balance the potential risks and benefits of any treatment plan. Opioids pose a number of potential risks beyond misuse and addiction, including suppression of respiratory drive, constipation, sleep apnea, and endocrine dysfunction. But, in the face of an individual in pain, doing nothing can also carry risk. For example, consider the case of a 76-year-old woman who came into an emergency room after a motor vehicle accident with rib fractures. Twenty-four hours later, her pain was causing her to suppress coughing and splint her breathing, leading to inadequate ventilation and raising her risk of pneumonia and death. This is an extreme example of how under-treatment of pain may be lethal.

Although most cases aren't this clear or dramatic, ongoing pain undermines quality of life and slowly erodes a person's physical, emotional, and spiritual wellbeing. Both directly (via inappropriate activation of stress-related mediators) and indirectly (by inducing inactivity, insomnia, anxiety, depression, and many other forms of physical and mental deterioration), pain compromises both mind and body. Uncontrolled chronic pain also undermines the management of any preexisting chronic condition, such as diabetes, cardiovascular disease, and psychiatric conditions such as anxiety or depressive disorders. Chronic pain in combination with depression increases the risk of suicide.

Looking at the complete landscape of pain and its collateral damage, it is clear that the decision whether or not to treat pain offers clinicians no risk-free option. If the overall risk to the patient associated with a given treatment is greater than the risk of withholding that treatment, then that treatment cannot be chosen. Among treatments that pose less risk than

> *All patients complaining of pain deserve adequate evaluation and treatment based on careful consideration of risks and benefits to the patient.*

withholding treatment, those treatments with the least risk and greatest benefit are the clear choices. Too often however, prescribers must use medical judgment in weighing risks and benefits without complete clarity on either side. Although prescribers should not feel compelled to use any treatment modality (including opioid analgesics), the risk of non-treatment or under-treatment must always be factored into any pain-management decision.

Non-treatment or under-treatment of pain can also pose risks to clinicians. In a few cases, physicians have been successfully sued for not treating pain aggressively. For example, the 2001 Bergman vs. Eden Medical Center case involved a physician who was found guilty of "elder abuse" arising from allegedly under-prescribing pain medication.[24] The jury brought a $1.5 million verdict against this physician and was a single vote away from levying much higher damages. This case led the California legislature to pass a law requiring the State Medical Board to publicly declare its policies on how it investigates physicians in pain management cases, and requiring all California physicians to have mandatory CME credits on pain management and end-of-life care. Another California case in which a physician was accused of elder abuse for under-treating pain was settled out of court for an undisclosed sum. In that case, the Medical Board formally and publicly sanctioned the physician for under-treatment of pain. Even though such cases represent rather extreme situations, these legal precedents sound a warning that there are potential risks to physicians associated with under-treating pain.

This does not imply, of course, that all patients must be treated aggressively with opioids or any other specific treatment. It simply means that all patients complaining of pain deserve adequate evaluation and treatment based on careful consideration of risks and benefits to the patient. With transparent documentation that clearly supports the rationale for treatment decisions, prescribers should feel comfortable that they have done their best to provide appropriate patient care while meeting their fiduciary obligations as "officers of the public health." Clinicians who withhold a treatment, based on an assessment that the treatment's risk is not in the patient's best interest, should not be seen as under-treating. On the contrary, it should be viewed as a sign of high quality, patient-oriented care.

## Exceptions

It's not always possible to obtain a thorough history or risk assessment for a patient. In the emergency department, the operating room, at night or on weekends, a prescriber may not always be able to verify the patient's history and past medical treatment. In such circumstances, clinicians must balance the need for vigilance about risks such as potential addiction or diversion with the risk associated with delayed treatment of the patient's pain. As with most treatment decisions, an approach based on risk versus benefit must determine the appropriate response. Clinicians are commonly faced with risks associated with treating as well as with withholding treatment. Too often, it is impossible to know which risks are most likely and the clinician must make choices that range from treating based on the avoidance of suffering and acceptance of potential risk for misuse, or withholding a particular treatment because of potential misuse and acceptance of the risk that the patient might suffer unnecessarily. Such decisions must be based on the short- and long-term impact of the treatment, its duration, and the potential for diagnosing an adverse outcome were it to occur. For example, it might be perfectly acceptable practice in the case of a complaint of pain in the emergency room to prescribe small amounts of an opioid analgesic that would get the patient through to the following day until a clinician with a longitudinal relationship with the patient is available to follow up. The potential harm from under-treated pain, weighed against the limited potential harm of a few opioid pills, may support this determination.

## Summary

Effective patient evaluation, selection, and assessment involves all of the elements of a traditional patient workup, with additional attention to pain history; prior analgesic approaches, therapies, or interventions; examination of mental illness; assessment of substance misuse risk, including personal and family history of substance abuse and substance abuse treatment; and review of relevant records, including a report from the prescription drug monitoring system if one is available.

Three steps can improve the quality of a history taken from a patient in pain: (1) take control of your time; (2) focus on the patient, not the pain; and (3) use reflective listening skills. Be alert to signs that a patient is minimizing his or her pain. Bear in mind that when considering use of a controlled substance in pain treatment, risk of misuse is always a possibility and must be assessed. Although the vast majority of patients are not abusing drugs, clinicians must remain vigilant in their attention to this possibility. It is fundamental that clinicians recognize that the risk of non-treatment with an opioid medication must always be factored into any pain management decision; not treating pain is often not a "safe" option. All patients complaining of pain deserve adequate evaluation and treatment based on careful consideration of risks and benefits.

# Chapter 3
## *Creating a Treatment Plan*

Once a patient has been evaluated and accepted as a candidate for treatment, and after adequate informed consent is obtained for such treatment (see Chapter 4 for discussion of patient consent and agreements), a written plan for implementing the treatment should be drafted. Such plans typically begin by stating the objectives of treatment, and this initial component deserves careful consideration. Because measuring pain is inherently subjective, setting pain relief as the sole outcome of treatment establishes an outcome that will be impossible to measure objectively. Indeed, the very notion of "pain relief" contains the hidden assumption that it's possible and desirable to "relieve" pain completely.

In fact, everyone lives at certain times with some kind of physical and/or emotional pain or discomfort. Few people are completely pain free for long! In fact, the rare cases of people with a congenital inability to feel pain demonstrate (usually tragically) the profound disadvantages of a life with "zero pain."

Ironically, the traditional 0 to 10 pain scale used so often in clinical care perpetuates this misconception by implying that the ideal or attainable condition is "zero pain." It's a small leap from a 0-10 to scale to doctors and their patients assuming that the goal of pain treatment is the elimination of pain. But even setting the primary goal as pain reduction may miss an essential point: the sensation of pain is not the only important variable associated with a patient's complaint of pain and may not be the most important feature of the overall presentation. A critically important part of understanding pain—and a key to formulating an effective treatment plan—is to look at pain as an alarm system that may either be functioning properly to warn of harm or ongoing healing, or a disturbed system that is functioning abnormally.

*The sensation of pain may not be the most important feature of the overall presentation.*

Cases involving chronic pain may not be as clear cut as the example given earlier where we had an acute injury (rib fracture) and an objective target as an outcome of treatment (improved breathing). Patients with chronic pain undoubtedly suffer, but the cause of the pain and objective outcomes by which to measure treatment may not be immediately clear. Although we can empathize with a patient's suffering, we cannot know for sure how much pain the patient is actually experiencing, or the degree to which that pain may be relieved. Moreover, people differ widely in their pain tolerance. Our knowledge of a patient's subjective pain experience, therefore, is fundamentally limited. Are people who rate their pain as 9 on a 10-point scale, but who have no evidence of any negative impact of the pain on their overall life, in more pain than people who rate their pain as 6 but who have been unable to sleep, have become despondent, and cannot work because of their pain? Although the subjective experience of the pain is an important factor in the patient's suffering, only the functional impact of the pain can be used to create objective treatment goals. This chapter reviews how to create effective treatment plans based on this perspective.

## From Analgesia to Function: A Necessary Paradigm Shift

To be most effective, the objectives of any treatment plan should go considerably beyond analgesia or improving uni-dimensional pain intensity scores. Rather, outcome objectives should encompass a broader, function-based paradigm that targets the collateral damage of pain on various aspects of the patient's life. This approach offers the following tangible advantages:

- Treatment goals become more objective and verifiable (rather than relying on subjective reports alone).
- Individual differences among patients, both in terms of pain tolerance and functional goals, are respected.
- An individualized evidence base is created for making appropriate risk-benefit decisions on pain treatment options.
- Prescribing decisions (including decisions to wean a patient from a drug regimen) are tied to multidimensional outcomes, many of which may be objectively demonstrated to the clinician and the patient.

Most important, a function-based treatment strategy is the best way to maximize patients' quality of life and minimize the burden of their pain. Chronic pain diminishes function and erodes the foundations of daily life, such as physical activity, concentration, emotional stability, interpersonal relationships, and sleep. This can, in turn, degrade role function at work or in the home, which can lead to depression, anxiety, insomnia, and even suicide among other comorbidities.

Pain is an alarm that vividly grabs our attention. Anyone who has experienced severe pain knows how it demands our attention—multitasking is nearly impossible for someone in severe pain. Ongoing chronic pain makes it difficult to attend to the activities that make life worth living. Our ability to function is disrupted, and ultimately, may be disastrously impaired. Since persistent pain decreases function, relieving pain should therefore improve function. Simply "feeling better," without measurably improving functioning in some aspect of the patient's life, is an insufficient outcome. Framing the treatment goal solely around "feeling better" also leaves the clinician with no objective evidence by which to gauge the efficacy of therapy and justify potential risks associated with the treatment.

Using objective, function-based treatment goals is a paradigm shift for many clinicians who may have been trained to focus almost exclusively on reducing or eliminating a patient's pain intensity rating. But reducing a patient's pain score from, say, 9 to 3 is only one piece of a much larger puzzle. Clinicians must also be mindful of the potential collateral costs of pain reduction with opioids, including sedation, constipation, endocrine effects, limitations on driving, and additional security responsibilities relating to having controlled substances in the home. Depending only on subjective outcomes can lead a physician to overlook evidence that a medication is ineffective or is producing side effects that are reducing quality of life. In some cases, pain may be relieved while the patient's functioning deteriorates. Possible reasons for a decline in function include:

- Exacerbation of a comorbid condition
- Side effects
- Use of analgesic medications for secondary purposes such as sleep or anxiety rather than pain
- Misuse or addiction

Using a function-based approach when creating a treatment plan allows a physician an optimal window from which to judge if a medication's side effects are presenting risks that outweigh the medication's benefits. In addition, basing a treatment plan on functional goals makes it harder for patients to mislead clinicians (and themselves) about their treatment outcomes.

## Functional Goals In a Treatment Plan

Creating a treatment plan based on functional goals makes some pre-scribers uneasy. It can be difficult to navigate the clinical landscape when a patient's subjective report of improvements in pain intensity are weighed against objective evidence that functional gains have not been achieved—or, worse, that actual harm is taking place. But clinicians fre-quently encounter analogous situations in other areas of medical prac-tice. For example, if a diabetic also has problems with chronic vasculitis, corticosteroids may effectively ease some of his or her symptoms. But corticosteroids, among other risks, worsen glucose control with seri-ous consequences in a diabetic. Diabetic patients who ask that they be chronically maintained on corticosteroids because the drugs make them

**CASE STUDY**

Mike was a 38-year-old construction worker with lumbar disc injury. After laminectomy and fusion surgery, the expected bone regrowth didn't occur, and the fusion surgery was repeated. This fusion appeared to work, but he continued to be in pain. Several nerve block procedures failed to provide relief.

After several housebound months, Mike sought help at a nearby pain center. He lacked energy, slept only in his reclining lounge chair, and was often irritable and short-tempered with his wife and children. He complained that the hydrocodone he was prescribed wasn't working anymore. His wife reported that Mike had used vari-ous non-medical drugs in the past and currently consumed alcohol a few times each week.

His physician negotiated a realistic function-based treatment plan for Mike. His initial goals were to sleep in his bed again, attend a meeting at his son's elementary school, enroll in a pain support group, and begin a program of gentle but long-term physical therapy. Four weeks later Mike had titrated up his opioid dose as prescribed.

"The medication is really working, Doc," Mike reported. "My pain's gone from an 8 to a 2 most of the time."

But under questioning it became clear that Mike had not actu-ally made progress. He was still sleeping in the lounge chair. He feel better challenge the physician to make a rational clinical decision weighing the risks and benefits in the wider context of overall functioning. No reputable physician would accommodate such a request except under highly select circumstances (e.g., end-of-life care where comfort is the principle goal of treatment). Most would recognize that the risks outweigh the benefits. The physician is forced to say, "I'm sorry, but I can't give you this medication even though it makes you feel better because it's going to harm you in the long run."

The clinician's response to a patient who continues using an opioid medication, but whose quality of life is unchanged or actually worsens, must be the same: "This treatment is not working well. Let's find a more effective way to both control your pain and improve the quality of your day-to-day life (or help you become more functional)."

As this case study illustrates, some patients may report large changes in their pain score even as their quality of life erodes.

missed the school meeting. He had only seen the physical therapist once. He also wasn't sleeping well, even though he felt drowsy most of the time.

The physician realized that the sedation Mike was experiencing was interfering with his progress toward functional goals.

After considerable patient education and negotiation, Mike agreed to taper off the opioid and try a new regimen of a non-addicting stimulant in the morning and a sedating medication for the evening. This normalized his sleep/wake cycles and left him with more energy during the day. He used non-opioid analgesics for his pain.

Two weeks later, Mike had attended two meetings of a chronic pain support group, and his wife reported that he had been regularly attending physical therapy. Four weeks later Mike looked relaxed and alert. His pain was not gone; he said it varied from about a 3 to a 5 (out of 10) from day to day. But he said he could live with that. He was moving around, making slow but steady progress in physical therapy, and becoming socially active. He was benefiting from a positive feedback loop: a relatively minor reduction in pain led to real improvements in function. This, in turn, further reduced the importance of pain in his life, which facilitated increased function in his daily routine.

This is an example of treatment success with a modest pain score reduction. In fact, a 20% reduction in a pain score (i.e., two points on the standard pain scale) may be a perfectly acceptable goal when it produces significant functional benefits for a patient. Cleeland and Ryan (1994) showed how increasing pain severity tracks with decreased function, starting with impacts on enjoyment, work, and mood at moderate pain levels, and proceeding to disruptions in physical activity, sleep, and relationships as pain severity increases.[25] The key point is that seemingly modest reductions in pain can translate into significant functional improvements as pain rating declines. A patient told that a specific treatment will reduce his or her pain by 20 percent may be unimpressed by this goal—because, like many clinicians, they focus solely on pain intensity rather than its impact. But, in fact, this change may halt a pattern of progressive functional loss.

Note that a single pain score may be important to patients as a quantitative yardstick with which to effectively communicate with their healthcare providers, but pain is so subjective that a single value on a single visit is much less useful than monitoring pain scores over time. If the treatment outcome is framed in terms of reclaimed function through a modest reduction on the pain scale, patients may be more likely to appreciate this as a major positive outcome and commit to this treatment goal.

Although a treatment plan may include reductions in pain scores, such reductions should not be used in isolation or as the sole determinant of treatment success for a chronic condition.

## Function and Controlled Substances

Switching to a function-based paradigm for treatment plans has particular value in the area of controlled substances because functional goals help to differentiate a patient who is truly addicted from one who looks addicted, but is not. This differentiation is grounded in the principle that addiction and pain lead to dysfunction, while pain relief should improve function. When given adequate pain relief, persons in chronic pain can gain or maintain

*Addiction and pain lead to dysfunction, while pain relief should improve function.*

function in their lives. Addiction, on the other hand, involves drug use that causes dysfunction in one or more spheres of a person's life.

Addicts have a disease that impairs their ability to control or modulate their use of a drug despite the dysfunction and harm it causes. In the setting of active addiction, function does not improve with exposure to the drug. Although analgesic trials that do not lead to functional improvement are often because of something other than addiction or misuse, the lack of functional improvement always indicates a problem with the treatment or some other facet of the patient's life that deserves attention. At the very least, in cases where analgesic trials do not lead to functional improvement, re-evaluation should occur, using a differential diagnosis that considers the possibilities of substance misuse, diversion, or addiction.

Reduced functioning may be rooted in function-limiting side effects, such as sedation, or may be caused by untreated affective disorders that are commonly associated with chronic pain. Sometimes, however, the manifestation of dysfunction will represent addiction, diversion, or misuse—a distinction that may be difficult to make without objective measures. Putting functional goals at the heart of a treatment plan can shed valuable light on the sometimes confusing presentations of patients in pain. (The subject of addiction versus pseudo-addiction is covered in more detail in Chapter 6: Periodic Review and Monitoring.)

## Putting a Function-Based Approach Into Action

You don't need expensive interventions or high-tech diagnostics to embark on a function-based treatment plan. All you need is a pen, paper, and the information you've gleaned from your patient. The functional goals of a treatment plan must be achievable and realistic. Progress in restoring function is usually slow and gains are usually incremental. Chronic pain is often marked by long-standing physical and psychological deconditioning, and recovery requires

> *"What do you hope to do with this treatment that you can't do now?"*

reconditioning that may take weeks, months, or years. Clinicians must educate patients about this reality so that they expect a marathon, not a sprint, on the road to recovery. Experience shows that if a patient can achieve one goal, his or her motivation and attitude improves, making the next goal that much easier to achieve. As with other life pursuits, "The key to success is success."

Here, for example, is how a set of functional goals could be set up for "Mike," the construction worker featured in the case study earlier in this chapter. Although Mike was initially focused exclusively on pain relief, an astute clinician would, after sufficient medical evaluation for any treatable conditions, search for a strategy to improve his activity level, restore his self-esteem, and rebuild his quality of life. Often the best place to start is with a simple yet important question: "What do you hope to do with this treatment that you can't do now?" Sometimes patients won't know how to answer at first because they are not used to thinking in terms of functional goals. They might say, "I don't know . . . I just want to feel better, that's all."

As just explained, although understandable, this response does not help to develop a set of realistic functional goals and some "hard" measures by which to evaluate outcomes. As we saw, after more discussion, Mike decided he wanted to sleep in his bed again instead of the reclining chair, and he wanted to be more involved at his son's school. To create some measures of progress toward these goals Mike agreed to bring records from his support group and have his wife confirm his progress in the other areas. This gave Mike and his clinician the start of a road map by which to measure progress and an evidence trail on which to base treatment decisions.

This approach also lays the foundation for making decisions about changing the course of treatment, or even terminating treatment, if goals are not met, adverse effects outweigh benefits, or in rare cases of deceit or diversion. For persons intent on abusing prescription drugs, participating in a function-based treatment plan presents some formidable hurdles. Such individuals may seek care elsewhere rather than undertake the effort of participating in a game of "functional outcomes charade."

Table 5 illustrates some simple functional goals and ways they might be verified.

When validation requires a report from a spouse, partner, family member, or friend, it may be useful (if the patient gives consent) to have that person accompany the patient to follow-up visits. Of course, no validation scheme is 100-percent foolproof. Somebody determined to fool a clinician will find a way. But experience suggests that dysfunctional or deceptive patients reveal themselves at some point—and repeated requests for evidence of improved function unmask deception earlier in the course of treatment. Deceitful patients rarely are able to

**TABLE 5. EVIDENCE FOR FUNCTIONAL GOALS**

| Functional Goal | Evidence |
| --- | --- |
| Begin physical therapy | Letter from physical therapist |
| Sleeping in bed as opposed to lounge chair | Report by family member or friend (either in-person or in writing) |
| Participation in pain support group | Letter from group leader |
| Increased activities of daily living | Report by family member or friend |
| Walk around the block | Pedometer recordings or written log of activity |
| Increased social activities | Report by family member or friend |
| Resumed sexual relations | Report by partner |
| Returned to work | Pay stubs from employer or letter confirming the patient is off of disability leave |
| Daily exercise | Gym attendance records or report from family member or friend |

continue faking functional improvement, particularly if their general level of function is, in fact, decreasing.

But the purpose of validating treatment goals is not simply to detect misuse of prescription drugs—though it can certainly help in that area. The main purpose of putting "teeth" into a functional goal-oriented plan is to motivate patients to achieve their goals, reclaim collateral losses, and thereby improve quality of life. In the process, the clinician obtains the information needed to determine whether or not a given course of treatment is working. The evidence you request will vary with the patient, and your clinical judgment will dictate what evidence you require, for how long, and to what degree it will be weighted in your assessment of treatment success.

Remember that the patient is largely responsible for his or her therapeutic outcomes, and part of this responsibility is to provide you with evidence of his or her progress. Meeting this part of the prescribing agreement is a functional outcome in and of itself. Clinicians cannot be cast in the ongoing role of private investigators; patients must partner with their treater for the system to work. If a patient is unable to document or achieve the progress outlined in the plan, this is a failed functional outcome that suggests reassessment of the plan and possible readjustment of goals.

Functional goals should be revisited, and if needed, recalibrated at regular intervals.

## Components of an Effective Treatment Plan

A function-based treatment paradigm offers both the clinician and patient guidance through the often murky terrain of chronic pain management. What constitutes function is not preset and functional outcomes require an understanding of what has been lost, what of most value can be regained, and a willingness to look for a path forward. A patient in acute pain may simply need pain medication to improve breathing as measured by incentive spirometry, whereas a patient at the end of life may need an increase or reduction in opioid medication or different pain relievers to reduce sedation and enable meaningful conversations with loved ones. The details of the functional outcomes plan must and should be left to the patient and treating clinician to determine. In my experience, this does not necessarily require lots of time. Start with the introductory question: "What do you hope to do with treatment that you can't do now?" As you integrate this approach into your practice, keep these principles in mind:

- Elimination of all pain (i.e., "zero" pain) is usually neither possible nor desirable.
- A patient's pain score is just one of many variables related to his or her overall status and potential for recovery.
- Treatment goals should not be set primarily in the form of changes in pain scores.
- Seemingly minor pain-score reductions may actually correlate with major gains in reclaimed function.
- Functional goals must be set collaboratively between patient and clinician, be realistic and achievable, be meaningful to the patient, and be verifiable.
- Functional goals must be revisited and recalibrated at regular intervals.
- Because each patient's values and the functions he or she desire in life vary, each patient will have a unique set of functional treatment endpoints.
- Include as part of any treatment plan an up-front discussion of potential benefits as well as side effects, especially constipation, which are best addressed in a pro-active manner.
- Educate patients about the full range of issues surrounding safe use, storage, and disposal of opioids. (See Chapter 8 for a complete discussion of these issues.)

Although using functional outcomes may add some work to the start of a treatment plan, it will pay dividends over time. As noted above, a functional plan need not be onerous or complex. On the contrary, a commonsense and individualized approach can result from asking simple questions, respecting the patient's values, and targeting goals that are important to the patient, starting with the most attainable and progressing over time to greater challenges. Goals and progress must be periodically assessed, using the results to determine the direction of future care. At some point, patients may plateau at a certain level of function, and the clinician, in consultation with the patient, will have to use his or her clinical judgment to determine whether this is acceptable or whether changes are needed. Even after a plateau of stable medications balanced by stable functioning has been reached, ongoing periodic review with follow-up functional assessments is necessary in order to detect changes over time.

## Planning for Potential Treatment Discontinuation

No therapy is guaranteed to succeed. Responsible prescribers, therefore, must be as willing to stop a therapy as to start one. Clarity around starting and stopping treatment is important because, as we have seen, opioids are not curative, have no standard term of treatment or typical time course and are associated with substantial risks. Both the prescriber and the patient should be prepared for all potential aspects of the treatment experience. Thus, a strategy for terminating opioid therapy (i.e., an exit plan) is part of the overall treatment plan and is always best prepared in advance.

The treatment plan should anticipate potential discontinuation points of treatment, even if this part of the plan is never implemented. Discontinuation may be required for many reasons, including:
- Pain is no longer a problem because of resolution of the previously painful condition.
- The experience of intolerable side effects.
- Lack of adequate response to a medication in terms of either pain relief or functional improvement.
- Evidence of non-medical or inappropriate use of the medications.

Patients should also be fully educated about all of the known benefits and risks of the chosen treatment. With opioids, this includes the realities of tolerance and physical dependence and the potential resulting need to taper the medication slowly to avoid withdrawal. They must also be educated about the possibilities that opioids may either be ineffective or have intolerable adverse effects including, but not limited to, the appearance of aberrant behaviors, misuse, or addiction. Treatment planning must include this type of education and can be most expeditiously handled by preparing in advance for the patient in chronic pain. Often, this kind of education can be offered through either informed consent forms or prescriber/patient agreements. (These subjects are covered extensively in Chapter 4.)

It may be helpful to include explicit descriptions of what is considered treatment "success" and treatment "failure." Why the drug is being started and why it may be discontinued is critical information for any patient to know in choosing to start long-term opioid therapy. It's usually easy to discuss the potential benefits for treatment but more difficult to review reasons for discontinuation, such as egregious, intractable, aberrant behavior.

Regulators will want patients to be aware of what will occur in the event that inappropriate use of a prescription is discovered. In the case of clear evidence of diversion, treatment must be suspended. Medical judgment, however, must be used to determine if other treatments might be helpful or viable in the patient's care. In a case of known opioid misuse, some clinicians may feel that continued pain treatment may be justified if done with intensified monitoring, patient counseling, and careful documentation of all directives, heightened risk management, and close attention to functional outcomes. *It must be stressed, however, that for most patients who have demonstrated clear signs of drug misuse or addiction, the level of vigilance and risk management needed for safe continuation of long-term opioid dosing often exceeds the abilities and resources of the average prescriber.* This must be considered before continuing opioid therapy in the face of evidence of misuse, diversion, or addiction. Before deciding whether to continue prescribing opioids in such cases, clinicians should seek consultation from, or referral to, specialists with greater knowledge and expertise in dealing with substance abuse and addiction.

SAMHSA offers many useful resources for clinicians treating patients at risk for substance abuse and addiction, including:

- Substance Abuse Treatment Facility Locator at http://findtreatment. samhsa.gov
- Treatment Improvement Protocol (TIP 54) for Managing Chronic Pain in Adults With or in Recovery From Substance Use Disorders can be downloaded or ordered at: http://store.samhsa.gov/shin/content//SMA12-4671/SMA12-4671.pdf
- A web-based resource for clinicians who wish to combine medication and behavioral therapies at http://dpt.samhsa.gov

## Summary

Chapter 3 explored how to create effective treatment plans for patients in pain. In formulating a plan, it's important to focus well beyond pain relief. Complete evaluation and planning means looking beyond pain signals to the effects that those signals have on physical and psychosocial functioning. Outcomes are best objectified with improved functioning in multiple aspects of an individual's life. The process starts with the question: "What do you hope to do with this treatment that you can't do now?" Switching to a function-based paradigm provides a way to differentiate a patient who is succeeding with an analgesic treatment from someone who is not or who may be abusing, diverting, or addicted to a medication. Attention should be paid to even small reductions in the pain score, since they may correlate with extremely significant improvements in reclaimed function. Sustained success will require that functional goals are revisited and recalibrated at regular intervals by both doctor and patient. Moreover, the planning process must involve patient education around all relevant aspects of the medication, including safe use, storage, disposal, and the terms of ongoing prescribing and possible discontinuation.

# Chapter 4
## Documentation, Informed Consent, and Patient Agreements

Documentation and informed consent are vital to the management of any patient's pain, but particularly when controlled substances are used as part of pain management. Not only is clear, consistent, and detailed documentation part of "best practices," it is also necessary for reliable and legitimate assessment of the effectiveness of any treatment regimen. Documentation provides a transparent and enduring record of a clinician's rationale for a particular treatment. The focus in this chapter is on how to create and maintain the most useful and effective record for the benefit of both the patient and the clinician.

Given the impossibility of remembering the details of all the patients' care in a busy practice, a clear written record is the only way to recall the key elements of treatment and to spot trends over time—including progress toward functional goals, severity of side effects, or subtle changes in patient demeanor or affect. In the event the need arises to refer a patient to another clinician, careful documentation will enable optimal continuity of care.

Everybody wins when clinical decision-making is as shared and transparent as possible. Since risk management is a critical component of pain management, documenting the risk-benefit analysis as well as the risk management plan and course will be important components of the medical record for medical colleagues and for regulators. Put simply, this means creating records that accurately reflect how risks and benefits were considered, how the risk-benefit analysis for a particular patient was applied, and how it played out over time. This means documenting not only the basic care plan but the decision-making process and the rationale behind specific courses of treatment. Remember that both treating and not treating involve risks, so prescribers cannot avoid managing risks. Considering the risks and benefits of any treatment is a cornerstone of clinical practice, but many of us do not emphasize this in our clinical notes.

Many computerized systems are now available for the acquisition, storage, integration, and presentation of medical information. Most offer advantages that will benefit both patients and prescribers, such as records that are kept up to date, and the instant availability of information relevant to prescribing or treatment. In the future, even more sophisticated information systems may become available that include customized and automated patient-education and patient-assessment tools, as well as tools for collecting, analyzing, and utilizing outcomes data. Such systems offer the promise of greatly improving patient outcomes and patient satisfaction.

Although automation can help, clear documentation is not dependent on electronic record-keeping; it merely requires a commitment to creating clear and enduring communication in a systematic fashion. Good documentation can be achieved with the most elaborate electronic medical record systems, with paper and pen, or with dictated notes.

## Elements of Effective Documentation

As a broad guide, six basic elements of a patient's care should be documented in writing: (1) assessment, (2) education, (3) treatment agreement and informed consent, (4) action plans, (5) outcomes, and (6) monitoring.

Each clinician has to use his or her judgment to determine how much each element of documentation should be emphasized and how often it should be repeated. Each of these elements should at least be part of initial evaluations and should be considered for periodic updating. Regardless of the system used for documentation, detailed, readily available, and transparent medical records should cover the following areas:

- Medical history and physical examination
- Diagnostic and laboratory test results and therapeutic outcomes
- Prior evaluations and consultations
- Records of past treatment outcomes, including indicators of benefit such as functional outcomes, and indicators of risk such as adverse effects
- Medications (including date prescribed, type, dosage, strength, and quantity)
- Pain intensity levels
- Subjective complaints of the patient
- Objective findings related to subjective complaints, including impact on functioning and quality of life

- Diagnostic impressions, and potential treatment options
- Treatment objectives
- Discussion of risks and benefits
- Informed consent
- Instructions and agreements
- Plans for periodic review of treatment, including adverse effects, functional goals, and any other outcomes that reflect benefits or problems with the treatment

## Informed Consent

Informed consent is a fundamental part of planning for any treatment, but it's critically important in long-term opioid therapy, given its potential risks. At its best, consent fortifies the clinician/patient relationship. The informed-consent process can be a cornerstone of a patient-centered, supportive relationship where the choice of long-term opioid therapy is made with full understanding of its benefits and risks, as well as clear knowledge of the responsibilities of the patient and the prescriber. A thorough informed-consent process can also serve as a formalized patient-provider agreement that gives a patient a clear understanding of the nature of the treatment they are embarking on, including anticipated risks and benefits. Patient-provider agreements do not have to serve as informed consent documentation, and those that do not meet the full requirements of the informed-consent process cannot be used in lieu of meaningful informed consent.

There are at least four fundamental questions a clinician must be able to answer with confidence when obtaining informed consent in the context of treatment with opioids:[26]

1. Does the patient understand various options for treatment?
2. Has the patient been reasonably informed of the potential benefits and risks associated with those options?
3. Is the patient free to choose among those options, free from coercion by the healthcare professional, the patient's family, or others?
4. Does the patient have the capacity to communicate his or her preferences—verbally or in other ways (e.g., if the patient is deaf or mute)?

Informed consent is required, both legally and morally, and being prepared for this part of treatment will greatly help the prescriber as well as the recipient of care. (Be sure to obtain legal advice as to what constitutes informed consent, and adequate documentation thereof, in the jurisdiction(s) in which you practice.) Documentation that ensures that at least these minimal requirements of proper informed consent have been met, and that the issues involved were discussed and agreed upon by the patient, may be accomplished several ways, including incorporation into a treatment plan, incorporation into a patient agreement, or as a separate document. Since the patient's informed consent must be acquired whenever long-term opioid therapy is initiated, it behooves clinicians to have the necessary material on hand and to set aside an appropriate amount of discussion time with patients. With thoughtful preparation, informed consent can be accomplished efficiently and can help the prescriber feel more assured that he or she has a knowledgeable patient partner who is prepared for the responsibilities ahead. Well-executed informed consent can also help the patient understand that he or she has a responsible and ethical partner who respects their autonomy and personal rights.

## Patient-Provider Agreements

Patient agreement to many types of treatment, such as use of an antibiotic or a medication for diabetes, is often implied and not formalized in the medical record. For complex medical treatments such as pain management, more explicit documentation may be necessary. Without some standardization, patient education or informed consent may be unintentionally omitted, and conscious or unconscious biases may affect clinical decisions. In some areas of practice, such as treatment with opioids, formalizing the terms of care at the outset of treatment may be optimal for both the patient and prescriber.

Patient-provider agreements in the context of long-term opioid therapy have been critiqued as potentially coercive, if not unethical.[27] There is little doubt that opioid treatment agreements have been misused by some practitioners to increase the power differential in favor of the prescriber and to unethically place patients in the position of having to agree to its terms or else lose an important component of their treatment (or even lose all treatment). Such misapplication of the treatment agreement is not only unacceptable, it is unlikely to serve the intended purpose of facilitating patient adherence.

While formalized patient-provider agreements have not been validated as improving treatment efficacy, they have been widely used by clinicians treating patients in pain and are recommended by regulators and many experts on treatment guidelines for long-term opioid therapy.[28] Patient-provider agreements pre-date long-term opioid therapies and have been used by clinicians managing patients with impulsive or distorted thinking, such as those in suicidal states or with borderline personality disorders. The widespread use of formalized agreements for long-term opioid therapy suggests that clinicians feel that this treatment has a higher-than-normal potential to become difficult and requires extra safeguards. Moreover, endorsement of treatment agreements in long-term opioid therapy by regulators suggests that they view this practice as enhancing safety. Recently, the Veterans Administration (VA) and U.S. Department of Defense (DoD), which manage America's largest health systems, chartered an expert multidisciplinary panel, including ethicists and legal experts, that undertook a 2-year systematic review of existing medical literature. In their evidence-based, clinical practice guidelines published in 2010, the VA and DoD concluded that opioid treatment agreements are a standard of care when prescribing long-term opioid therapy.[29]

The major advantages of written agreements are that they can:

- Start treatment on a positive note of mutual respect and partnership, clarity of purpose and process, and transparency.
- Engage patients in a collaborative education and decision-making process.
- Assist in framing expected outcomes with specific functional goals and clarify the clinician's and patient's roles and responsibilities in attaining these goals.
- Document acceptance of risks and benefits of treatment and the details of the risk management program.
- Document informed consent for a variety of treatment approaches.
- Offer an opportunity for the patient to see and understand all aspects of the prescriber's operation as it applies to his or her specific treatment, with time provided to answer all questions he or she might have.
- Serve as motivational reminders to the patient and caregivers of the specific goals that have been mutually agreed upon.
- Help avoid misunderstandings or distortions of understanding that may occur over long treatment time periods.

- Provide a foundation for subsequent decision-making about changes in medications if functional goals are not achieved, or discontinuation of treatment if problems arise.
- Enhance the therapeutic relationship between patient and prescriber by enabling clear communication and the setting of clear expectations about the responsibilities that patients and their caregivers have for safe use of opioids.

A written agreement should document all the major points you have covered and agreed upon with the patient. Some pain-management centers use an agreement with all patients as part of their standard practice, because selective use of these tools can be perceived by patients as introducing bias. Some programs have even proposed generalizing the practice to include a written agreement with all analgesic treatments, based on the belief that a clearly written understanding of the agreed-upon treatment plan helps to enlist patient buy-in, even in regimens that do not include opioids. Although opioid prescribing may include more risk-management and monitoring obligations than some non-opioid analgesic regimens, any treatment regimen carries some degree of benefit and risk, and hence may be enhanced by the use of a clear agreement at the time of commencing treatment. Regardless of whether or not a controlled substance is being prescribed, there are tangible advantages to incorporating risk education information into a clear and transparent agreement process written at a reading level consistent with average patient literacy rates (generally about a sixth- or seventh-grade reading level).

It is worth noting that the term "agreement" is perceived by many to be more acceptable than "contract"—though from a legal standpoint, any written or oral agreement between a prescriber and a patient may be essentially considered a "contract" with elements that could be deemed as binding (particularly for the prescriber). Be sure that the terms in any agreement you use are understood by your patient, and are acceptable, attainable, and consistent with your practice. Agreements should be "patient-centered" and emphasize the attainment of positive outcomes for the patient. Although agreements usually describe the responsibilities of the patient, the responsibilities of the clinician should be clearly detailed as well. It may be helpful to include family members or caregivers in the discussions surrounding such agreements, since such people often need as much information as the patient in order to maximize safe use of opioids.

Treatment agreements come in a multitude of variations, and while there is no one-size-fits-all agreement, there is little question that some can be stigmatizing, patronizing, pejorative, or even punitive. Such tools place the patient at a disadvantage, or undermine care. The process can be used to intimidate patients and justify patient abandonment. Clinicians should strive to craft agreements that avoid these difficulties and that serve their patients' best interests.[27] Thus, agreements should avoid:

- Placing all the burden of the agreement on the patient rather than sharing it between patient and clinician.
- Framing the agreement as a punishment for future crimes or difficulties, or in terms other than choices that serve the patient's best interests.
- Using language that is stigmatizing, dominating, or pejorative.
- Using coercion in any way.
- Imposing limitations for the clinician's convenience without clear and substantial benefit for the patient.
- Insisting on behaviors unrelated to actual use of medications (i.e., "you will be respectful of me and my staff" or "you will be on time for appointments").
- Suggesting that each patient will be treated in any way other that as an individual with individualized treatment decisions that are always based on the individual patient's best interest.
- Using the term "fired" to describe discontinuation of treatment.
- Threatening abandonment or suggesting that each patient will not have the benefit of individualized re-evaluation and continued access to other non-opioid pain relieving treatments that are safe and potentially effective for him or her.

## Components of an Effective Agreement

Although examples of standard treatment agreements or informed consent documents for opioid treatment are available at professional society websites, such as the American Academy of Pain Medicine (www.painmed.org), there are many variations of agreements that can be tailored for specific types of treatment. They can offer fixed language or include "open" areas to be filled in with specific and unique aspects of the patient's treatment plan. For example, a list of functional goals can be generated within an agreement (written in by hand or typed into a computer-based form or electronic medical record and printed out for signing). Clinicians may want to consider adding any of the following elements to their treatment agreements:

- Education about the risks and benefits of the agreed-upon treatment, including available alternatives to treat pain.
- Clarification of goals for treatment decisions.
- Explanation that the patient is being prescribed an opioid initially on a trial basis only.
- The clinician's responsibilities.
- Expectations around individualized goals and agreed-upon processes for documenting progress.
- Explanations of potential adverse outcomes such as addiction, tolerance, physical dependence, constipation, nausea, or itching.
- Need for the patient to inform the treating prescriber of relevant information (i.e., side effects, use of other medications, changes in condition, inability to meet agreed upon goals, history of substance misuse).
- Statement of time frame for which the agreement is in effect.
- Expectation of a single designated prescriber for all opioids, and a single designated pharmacy to fill these prescriptions.
- Requirements for including or communicating with additional healthcare providers (e.g., primary care physician, pharmacist, psychologist, physical therapist).
- Clarification of who receives the agreement, and where the agreement is kept.
- Statement of patient privacy rights.
- Relevant administrative policies.
- Explanation of circumstances in which treatment may be adjusted or discontinued (e.g., abusing medication, missed appointments, violating agreement, no improvement, tolerance, toxicity). This should include an explanation that, in most cases where opioids are not effective or have associated problems, discontinuing opioid treatment should not exclude the patient from being considered for all other safe and potentially helpful treatment options.
- Explanation of circumstances that would justify termination from the program, such as violence or situations where continuing in the program would no longer serve the patient's best interest. This should include a clear description of how the program will avoid abandoning the patient.

Written agreements involving any controlled substance should include the following additional elements:

- Patient responsibilities to avoid improper use of controlled substances (e.g., exceeding prescribed dose, seeking medication elsewhere, selling or sharing medication, stopping medication abruptly).
- The policy on replacing lost medication or changing prescriptions
- The policy on drug refills (e.g., phone allowances, mailing or faxing policy, normal office hours).
- The policy for random drug screens.
- Education about safe storage and disposal of medications.
- Pharmacy issues (e.g., one pharmacy, in-state pharmacy).
- Additional risks (e.g., interactions with other drugs, masking conditions, driving safety, misusing, pregnancy).
- Legal considerations, where applicable under state laws. (See Chapter 10 for details of legal considerations.)
- Additional information regarding specific medications (e.g., type prescribed: long-acting, generic brands).

Written agreements are only effective to the extent that they are clearly understood. This means written materials and spoken words must be targeted to the education level of each patient. One study analyzing the reading grade level of opioid agreements found that the documents were at or above college reading level, although health literacy experts recommend that information be provided to patients at the sixth- to seventh-grade level or even below.[30, 31] This is even more significant for patients who do not speak English as a first language. English-language written agreements are commonly translated into Spanish, and translators for other languages can be provided for speakers of other languages to ensure patient understanding and effective informed consent.

Patients must be given the opportunity to ask questions, and prescribers should "check in" with patients to ensure they understand what they are being told. A treatment agreement that is simply handed to a patient without his or her input, or which is hastily explained and misunderstood by a patient, will not suffice. Patient agreements and/or consent forms should be reviewed carefully with patients and not treated as a mere formality to be buried in the chart. (Note that some parts or all of this task might be handled by trained "physician helpers" in the office—nurses, physician assistants, or other personnel.) Taking the time to make an agreement that fully informs all concerned transforms what could be a perfunctory document into a cornerstone of understanding about the agreed upon course of care, which may also contribute to treatment success.

Since most treatments carry some degree of risk, and more aggressive treatments usually carry greater risk, sharing these concerns and decisions about risk with patients is critically important. Patients, after all, ultimately take on the work of treatment adherence, tolerating possible side effects, and the challenges of achieving functional improvement. Moreover, they will bear the consequences of any adverse outcomes. A paternalistic approach, where the prescriber is the sole decision-maker, may result in half-hearted patient acceptance without investment or full commitment to the treatment. The lead architect of this treatment regimen—the prescriber—will then be responsible for failure to achieve desired outcomes. A better approach is to clarify the patient's appropriate responsibilities and to ensure that he or she clearly understands that treatment success or failure rests on his or her commitment and participation. It may be helpful for clinicians to view themselves as an expert advisor or consultant. The patient, meanwhile, may be best served by accepting the role of "chief executive officer" of his or her treatment regimen.

Effective communication and patient education are integral parts of "best practices" from both an ethical and legal standpoint. A patient who does not fully understand the potential risks and benefits of a procedure or treatment cannot be truly "informed" as required by both legal and the ethical guidelines for medical practice. Inadequate communication on the part of a prescriber and the failure to educate the patient about the treatment regimen can potentially destabilize the therapeutic relationship, disempower the patient, and leave the prescriber vulnerable to claims that the treatment would not have been accepted had its risks and benefits been fully understood.

## Universal Precautions

The phrase "universal precautions" originated in the field of infectious diseases and is increasingly used in pain management. The term refers to a standardized approach to the assessment and ongoing management of *all* a clinician's patients with pain. Just as it is impossible to predict if patients (or their body fluids) will harbor an infectious agent, it's impossible to predict with any degree of certainty which patients in pain will misuse prescription medications. Taking universal precautions against prescription opioid misuse with all patients (such as, treatment agreements, random drug screening, or screening instruments for risk of misuse) offers a broader safety net while avoiding potential disparities in care. Universal precautions also help meet requirements for informed consent, improve patient education and participation, and minimize overall risk. If logistical or financial constraints limit your ability to practice universal precautions, one alternative is to employ random screening only on high-risk patients or patients exhibiting aberrant behavior. Since even experts in addiction and pain medicine are fallible when predicting who is and is not at risk for opioid misuse, such approaches risk stigmatizing patients and creating disparities in care.

## Summary

Clear and transparent documentation is essential at every step of the process of delivering appropriate pain care. Moreover, complete documentation is essential to comply with state and federal laws governing prescription of controlled substances.

There are tangible advantages to creating a clear and enduring treatment agreement that incorporates informed consent language, statements of expectations, and patient education about the risks and benefits of treatment, as well as safe use and disposal of medications. Clinicians should strive to craft agreements that are fair, balanced, clear, and non-coercive and that promote informed participation and shared decision-making. A well thought out, written treatment agreement delineates the responsibility of the patient to the prescriber and the prescriber to the patient. In creating an agreement, be sure that the terms you use are completely comprehensible and attainable, and that no treatments or processes are listed that your practice does not actually provide. Prescriber/patient agreements must also be drafted at a reading level appropriate for a wide audience and written in a language your patients will comprehend. A patient who does not fully understand the potential risks and benefits of a procedure or treatment is not truly "informed" as required by both law and the ethical guidelines of medical practice. You can create treatment agreements using templates that are available online as a starting point or by creating one for the specific needs of your practice.

# Chapter 5
## *Initiating Treatment With Opioids*

When considering any new opioid prescription, clinicians should be certain that (1) all other potentially effective treatments that offer a more optimal risk to benefit profile have been considered or tried, (2) a complete evaluation has been performed and fully documented, (3) the patient's level of opioid tolerance has been determined, and (4) informed consent and agreement to treat has been obtained. At the outset, both the clinician and the patient should view a new opioid prescription as a short-term trial of therapy. The goal of the trial is to provide data that can guide decisions on the appropriateness of opioid medications in general and on the specific dose and formulation of medication. Such a trial might be as brief as a few hours or as long as several months.

Opioid selection, initial dosing, and titration must, of course, be individualized to the patient's health status, previous exposure to opioids, and treatment plan. Caution should be exercised when using opioids in patients with conditions that may be complicated by adverse effects from opioids, including COPD, CHF, sleep apnea, current or past alcohol or substance misuse, mental illness, advanced age, or patients with a history of renal or hepatic dysfunction. In addition, opioids should not be combined with other respiratory depressants, such as sedative-hypnotics (benzodiazepines or barbiturates) unless there is a specific medical and/or psychiatric indication for such a combination. In such cases, much more intensive monitoring is required.

A decision to continue opioid therapy after an appropriate trial should be based on careful review of the trial outcomes. Outcomes to consider include:

- Progress toward meeting therapeutic goals
- Changes in functional status
- Presence and nature of opioid-related adverse effects
- Changes in the underlying pain condition
- Changes in medical or psychiatric comorbidities
- Degree of opioid tolerance in the patient
- Identification of altered or aberrant behaviors, addiction, or diversion

As discussed earlier, agreement for treatment and informed consent are essential when initiating opioid therapy. Although informed consent is required for any treatment, prescribing long-term opioid therapy carries higher-than-normal potential for complications and risks, which many prescribers feel justifies extra safeguards. These safeguards might include the clinician's insistence that patients use a single prescriber or a single dispensing pharmacy, and implementation of toxicology screens or other risk management tools. Risk management must begin at assessment and be firmly in place at the time of initiating therapy.

## Dose Titration

Clinicians should initiate opioid-naïve patients or patients who have had only a modest previous opioid exposure of a low dose with a medication with a short duration of effect, and should carefully titrate upward to decrease the risk of opioid-related adverse effects. If you do not know whether the patient has recently been using opioids (either prescribed or non-prescribed), you should assume that the patient is opioid-naïve (i.e., not tolerant) and proceed as just described. Opioid tolerance must be demonstrated before prescribing any strength of extended-release (ER)/long-acting (LA) fentanyl and ER/LA hydromorphone and is usually prudent with any ER or LA opioid. The selection of a starting dose and manner of titration are clinical decisions that must be made on a case-by-case basis because of the many variables involved. As always, these decisions should be guided by a perspective that balances treatment benefits against treatment risks. In the setting of chronic pain, the adage "start low and go slow" holds many advantages. Some patients, such as frail older persons or those with comorbidities, may require an even more cautious therapy initiation. Short-acting opioids are usually safer for initial therapy since they have a shorter half-life and may be associated with a lower risk of inadvertent overdose related to sustained effects.

No direct evidence from randomized trials exists, however, that demonstrates the superiority of any particular opioid for initial therapy. Nonetheless, if opioids are to be started, common sense suggests that adversity is likely best avoided by starting with low dosages of an opioid with shorter durations of effect. Adverse effects will last longer when an LA opioid is prescribed than a short-acting formulation. Likewise, early use of as-needed dosing before committing to fixed, around-the-clock doses typically offers greatest safety. Nonetheless, there is insufficient evidence to guide exactly when its best to use short-acting versus LA opioids, or whether as-needed versus around-the-clock dosing is best. Well-conducted studies have not conclusively demonstrated more consistent control of pain or improved adherence associated with use of LA opioids with around-the-clock dosing. Although low dose, short-acting opioids may offer the greatest safety for initiating opioid therapy, clinicians must recognize that short-acting opioids are not intrinsically safer than other formulations. In fact, short-acting hydrocodone is widely misused and is involved in emergency room visits and toxic episodes. Many prescribers feel that hydrocodone's status as a schedule III opioid (when compounded with acetaminophen) should be changed to schedule II since the schedule III status suggests incorrectly that this drug is less risky or toxic than other opioids.

## Selecting an Appropriate Opioid

Opioids, as a class, comprise many specific agents available in a wide range of formulations. Short-acting formulations may be single agents or products that combine an opioid with a non-opioid analgesic, such as acetaminophen. Some ER/LA opioids have relatively long-durations of effect because of intrinsic pharmacological properties independent of how the drug is compounded (particularly methadone). Most, however, are formulated for prolonged duration of effect and thus the terms ER or sustained-release opioid may be synonymous with an LA opioid formulation. A given patient might be appropriate for LA only, short-acting only, or a combination of an LA opioid with a short-acting opioid for breakthrough pain. Clinicians must have a thorough knowledge of the specific characteristics of any ER/LA opioid product they prescribe, including the drug substance, dosage form/strength, dosing interval, key instructions, major drug interactions, use in opioid-tolerant patients, drug-specific adverse events, and relative potency compared to oral morphine.

LA opioids usually have a relatively slow onset of action (typically between 30 and 90 min.) and a relatively long duration of action (4 to 72 hours). These agents achieve their extended activity in various ways. Methadone and levorphanol have intrinsic pharmacokinetic properties that make their effects more enduring than many short-acting opioids. However, these analgesic effects are less pronounced than in most opioids that are formulated for sustained-release. LA agents such as controlled-release morphine, oxycodone, or transdermal fentanyl achieve their prolonged time course via a delivery system that is modified to slow absorption or to slow the release of the active ingredient. Methadone can be an effective opioid, but it must be prescribed carefully and with full knowledge of its highly variable pharmacokinetics and pharmacodynamics. (See a detailed discussion in Chapter 7.)

Short-acting opioids typically have rapid onset of action (10-60 min.) and relatively short duration of action (2-4 hours). They are used for intermittent pain or breakthrough pain that occurs against a background of a persistent level of pain.

Combination products join an opioid with a non-opioid analgesic, usually for use in patients with moderate pain. Typically, the non-opioid co-analgesic agent, such as acetaminophen or an NSAID, has a ceiling dose above which efficacy will plateau as risk for adverse effects increases. Acetaminophen may reach toxic levels at a dose of hydrocodone that is effective and well tolerated. Thus, these combination products are typically used for patients who are not expected to need substantial dose escalations. Using a combination product when dose escalation is required risks increasing adverse effects from the non-opioid co-analgesic, even if increase of the opioid dose is appropriate. For instance, if a patient is prescribed increasing dosages of a hydrocodone-acetaminophen medication, the acetaminophen may reach toxic levels while the increased dose of hydrocodone is effective and well tolerated. In such cases, using just the opioid component may be the best option. Unfortunately, at this time, no pharmaceutically manufactured single-agent option for hydrocodone is available, although clinical trials are underway as part of an effort to secure FDA approval for just such an agent. Single-agent formulations are available for other types of opioids, such as morphine, oxycodone, and hydromorphone.

See Appendix E for a listing of opioid medications with recommended starting doses and other valuable information.

Another consideration to bear in mind at the initiation of a course of opioid treatment is whether, or how, to provide for breakthrough pain episodes. This important topic is discussed fully in Chapter 6.

## Anticipating and Preventing Adversity

Although a well-crafted patient–provider agreement, an informed consent document, or both will advise patients of potential adverse events with opioids, clinicians should also review these issues verbally when initiating opioid therapy. In particular, patients should be advised about the likelihood of constipation and be provided with education and means of prophylaxis. The potential for other adverse events should also be discussed, including sedation, itching, gastro-intestinal upset, and enhancement of respiratory depression. Impairment of the ability to drive is a serious potential adverse effect that requires early consideration, patient education, and ongoing monitoring. (See Chapter 8 for more on educating patients about adverse events resulting from long-term opioid therapy.)

Some opioids have been found to enhance the neuromuscular-blocking action of skeletal relaxants, which could exacerbate the risk of respiratory depression. Since neuromuscular-blocking drugs are usually used in operating room settings and largely by anesthesiologists, this risk is unusual in a clinic setting. Likewise, a relationship between opioids and monoamine oxidase inhibitors (MAOIs) has long been established, particularly with the opioid meperidine. Combining meperidine, and more rarely, fentanyl or morphine, with an MAOI can lead to a potentially life-threatening reaction including seizure, fever, muscle rigidity, respiratory distress/depression, flushing, sweating, and unconsciousness. MAOI use in the United States, however, is increasingly rare because of the need for dietary restrictions and an unfavorable side-effect profile relative to newer agents. In patients using MAOIs, opioids should be avoided for at least 2 weeks after MAOI discontinuation. Clinicians should also be aware that since opioids are known to affect the release of antidiuretic hormone (ADH), they may interact with diuretics.

A new approach to reducing adverse events with opioids involves providing patients with intranasal naloxone to take home and use in case of overdose. This has proven valuable in some communities. "Project Lazarus" in Wilkes County, NC, for example, provided patients with take-home intranasal naloxone as a result of data showing that half of overdose deaths occurred in home settings. Preliminary data from the program show that the overdose death rate in the community decreased 38% between 2009 and 2010.[32] If these results are sustained and seen elsewhere, intranasal naloxone may become a more widely adopted component of long-term opioid therapy.

As part of responsible opioid prescribing, the FDA recommends that both prescribers and their patients report side effects to the FDA by calling a dedicated line: 1-800-332-1088, or by using an online form, available at: http://www.fda.gov/safety.

## Abuse-Deterrent and Other New Formulations

Recently, opioid manufactures have developed abuse-deterrent and tamper-resistant opioid formulations to reduce opioid misuse. Several different formulations have been developed. One incorporates an opioid antagonist into a separate compartment deep within a single capsule; crushing the capsule will release the antagonist and neutralize the opioid effect. The central opioid antagonist compartment is eliminated unchanged if the capsule is consumed normally without tampering. Another strategy is to modify the physical structure of tablets or incorporate compounds that make it difficult or impossible to liquefy, concentrate, or otherwise transform the tablets. To date, several compounds with these strategies have been approved by the FDA, but none have applied for abuse-resistant labeling. Clinicians should always warn patients that under no circumstances should an oral ER/LA opioid be broken, chewed, or crushed, and patches should not be cut or torn prior to use, since this may lead to rapid release of the opioid and could cause overdose or death.

Current abuse-resistant formulations discourage abusers from manipulating, concentrating, or otherwise changing the original formulation of the drug. Prescribers must remain aware, however, that the formulations do not prevent abusers or unintentional misusers from simply consuming too much of a medication. Moreover, it remains to be seen if these abuse- and tamper-resistance strategies will truly deter determined abusers and reduce misuse or diversion. We need long-term trials, longer clinical experience, or both to answer these questions. In the meantime clinicians must consider some issues related to these new formulations:

- Does the higher cost of these formulations pose challenges for patients and/or limit their accessibility?
- Are there any ethical issues related to prescribing abuse-deterrent formulations for some, but not all, patients?

Historically, transdermal preparations have been perceived as less vulnerable to misuse, but transdermal formulations have been tampered with and abused. A transdermal, 7-day duration formulation of buprenorphine was approved by the FDA in July 2010 for treatment of chronic pain. This drug is a partial μ opioid agonist that is used in its sublingual tablet and soluble film forms for opioid addiction treatment. It is marketed as buprenorphine/naloxone tablets and soluble films (Suboxone®), and buprenorphine without naloxone tablets (previously sold as Subutex® and also available as a generic. There is no soluble film form of buprenorphine without naloxone.) Forms of buprenorphine may have potential advantages as a lower-risk agent than full μ agonist opioid treatment medications. Nonetheless, reports have described increased levels of diversion and non-medical use of buprenorphine, including in forms smuggled into prison populations. There is little doubt that buprenorphine can be misused; whether or not it will offer advantages to full-opioid agonists remains to be determined.

## Summary

Clinicians must approach initiation of opioid therapy for pain management cautiously and with a clear understanding of the many variables that make it impossible to recommend standard starting doses or titration regimens. Initiating treatment with any opioid must always be based on evaluating associated risks and benefits, and requires an effective risk-management approach and plan. In patients without recent exposure to opioids, initial dosing and titration should be viewed by both patient and clinician as a trial, the results of which will determine whether further opioid therapy is warranted, and if so, which formulations and doses are likely to provide maximum benefits with minimal side effects.

Clinician experience and the needs of the specific patient must guide the selection of a particular opioid or its particular formulation. New abuse-deterrent formulations are intended to help curb some forms of misuse and diversion, although it is too early to determine their overall clinical impact.

# Chapter 6
## Management Strategies for Chronic Pain Patients: Periodic Review, Monitoring, and Discontinuation

If a trial of an opioid medication is deemed successful and opioid therapy is continued, periodic review and monitoring should be performed for the duration of treatment. The tests performed, questions asked, and evaluations made should be tailored to the patient as guided by the physician's clinical judgment. For example, a physical examination may or may not be required at each follow-up visit. (Check with your medical licensing board—some states may require a physical examination at each visit.) When opioids are prescribed, clinicians must attend to agreed-upon treatment outcomes and be alert to a wide range of potential adverse effects, ranging from physical side effects such as constipation or sedation to behavioral side effects such as mood changes, signs of drug craving or seeking, or impaired function in various domains of daily living. As part of routine practice, clinicians who prescribe opioids should perform medication reconciliation* at each patient visit.[33]

The intensity and frequency of monitoring is dependent on an assessment of the patient's risk for abuse, diversion, or addiction. Since every patient has some risk, an ongoing management plan is required in every opioid treatment. Tools and techniques similar or identical to those used during an initial assessment of a patient's risk can be used to re-assess or monitor risk on an on-going basis. (Appendix D presents links to common patient risk assessment tools.)

States vary in their requirements for intervals at which follow-up visits are required when controlled substances are prescribed. Although

---

* The American Medical Association (AMA) defines medication reconciliation as: "Making sense of a patient's medications and resolving conflicts between different sources of information to minimize harm and maximize therapeutic effects. It is an ongoing, dynamic, episodic, and team-based process that should be led by and is the responsibility of the patient's attending/personal physician in collaboration with other healthcare professionals. Medication reconciliation is essential to optimize the safe and effective use of medications. It is one element in the process of therapeutic use of medications and medication management for which physicians are ultimately held legally accountable."

federal law allows for a 90-day supply of prescriptions for patients receiving schedule II drugs (who are otherwise deemed safe to have this amount), state law can vary from 30 days to 6 months. In cases where state and federal law conflict, the most restrictive rule prevails. A clinician may deem it appropriate to monitor a low-risk patient on a stable dose of opioids less frequently than someone at greater risk. More frequent or intense monitoring may be appropriate for patients during the initiation of therapy or if the dose, formulation, or opioid medication is changed. Patients who may need more frequent or intense monitoring include:

- Those with a prior history of an addictive disorder, past abuse, or other aberrant use,
- Those in an occupations demanding mental acuity,
- Older adults,
- Patients with an unstable or dysfunctional social environment, and
- Those with comorbid psychiatric or medical conditions.

Management of chronic opioid therapy in high-risk patients was addressed in the 2009 American Pain Society/American Academy of Pain Medicine Clinical Guidelines for the Use of Chronic Opioid Therapy in Chronic Noncancer Pain:[28]

- Clinicians may consider chronic opioid therapy for patients with chronic noncancer pain and history of drug abuse, psychiatric issues, or serious aberrant drug-related behaviors only if they are able to implement more frequent and stringent monitoring parameters. In such situations, clinicians should strongly consider consultation with a mental health or addiction specialist.
- Clinicians should evaluate patients engaging in aberrant drug-related behaviors for appropriateness of chronic opioid therapy or need for restructuring of therapy, referral for assistance in management, or discontinuation of chronic opioid therapy.

Although it is possible to manage patients at high risk of abuse or addiction, it requires resources that are often well beyond those of the average prescriber. For instance, daily to weekly monitoring may be necessary for patients at very high risk for adverse outcomes. In cases when monitoring and management resources are inadequate to assure safety, refraining from prescribing may be the most supportable option and in the patient's best interest. You can find a good extended discussion of this subject in the Treatment Improvement Protocol from SAMHSA titled TIP 54: Managing Chronic Pain in Adults With or In Recovery from Substance Use Disorders (http://www.kap.samhsa.gov).

When considering a patient's level of risk and evaluating the structure and intensity of monitoring, clinicians should bear several points in mind:

- Even patients deemed to be "low risk" require a solid, ongoing risk management plan, because there is always *some* degree of risk involved with opioid pain medications.

- Despite a clinician's best efforts, patients may prove to be at greater risk than initially suspected, and risk management strategies may fail.

- The level of risk deemed acceptable will vary with the resources available to a clinician for keeping patients safe. For example, patients with respiratory dysfunction or sleep apnea may require resources beyond those available to a typical clinician, so the risk-benefit assessment of opioids would tilt away from the use of opioids unless additional resources were recruited.

## Reviewing Functional Goals

Monitoring a patient's progress toward a set of functional goals (as opposed to simply asking if he or she "feels better") requires a way of measuring progress (or lack thereof). This doesn't mean clinicians have to become private investigators, or that significantly more work is required, as long as the goals and means of verification are clearly set up from the beginning. The key is to work with patients to create a set of realistic treatment goals and a means of charting progress towards these goals. It is in the best interest of everyone involved in the prescribing process that the major responsibility for attaining those goals and presenting the evidence lies with the patient.

Patients in chronic pain often suffer collateral losses that are manifested through lost function and decreased quality of life. Reviewing a patient's functional losses and desired gains is an essential part of creating a treatment

*This pivotal question should now transform into "What can you do now that you could not do before treatment?"*

plan and is critical to establishing useful measures of progress on return visits. As reviewed in Chapter 3, functional goals should be objective, relatively easy to verify, and clear. They should also span as many domains of a person's life as possible: personal and social relationships, employment, physical activities, health, hobbies, and spiritual activities. Initial goals might have been set by the patient's answer to the simple question "What do you want to do with treatment that you can't do now?" This pivotal question should now transform into: "What can you do now that you could not do before treatment?" Sometimes goals will not be attained, requiring investigation and possible adjustments. On the other hand, if the goals *have* been attained, setting new goals is a good way to motivate further progress. For instance, if a patient, after three months of incremental improvement, has been able to return to swimming laps once a week, you might set a new goal of swimming two to three times a week. Conversely, if you've set an initial goal that was too ambitious, and the patient is becoming discouraged, you can revise the goal downward or change it altogether. Clinicians, in these situations, are analogous to a coach, providing both expert advice and counseling/motivation to support a patient's forward progress. Patients are like athletes training for a marathon (rather than a sprint). The clinician's aim is to create a set of attainable functional outcomes and set the stage for a new round of incrementally more ambitious goals. The key is to cultivate success, since this builds patient confidence and motivation. Setting goals that are too ambitious may lead a patient to believe he or she "failed," which can be a setback to both self-confidence and treatment progress.

A common dilemma for physicians is a patient who resists engaging in physical activity toward functional goals because he or she reports that any activity hurts too much. In such cases, rather than feeling forced to increase the dose of an opioid medication, the clinician might do better to step back and re-evaluate the functional goals. All patients—even those with end-stage disease—can engage in *some* kind of physical activity at least *some* time during the day. It may appear so minimal that it doesn't "count" as an "activity," but it may nonetheless be a starting point for a functional goal. It all depends on how you define function. Patients with a chronic pain condition may initially need an exceedingly gentle but regular exercise plan. This plan may require isolation or avoidance of specific painful areas until some degree of physical conditioning has been established. Again, patients in chronic pain require careful pacing and controlled, gradually-increasing, and frequent activity over sustained periods of time. If patients are not achieving their goals, especially if they are getting discouraged, consider affective disorders as a possible cause that may require specialized intervention, such as psychopharmacology, or referral to a therapist for cognitive-behavioral treatment.

The patient who says that he or she can't exercise because of pain may simply be signaling that their exercise is too intense or that they fear injury, increased pain, or even losing their identity as being "disabled." These myriad psychological barriers to an upward cycle of improvement are beyond the therapeutic reach of prescription drugs or nerve blocks, and are reminders of the importance of a team approach to integrated behavioral and rehabilitative pain management.

Almost all patients, however, can find some physical activity that does not cause pain. Although reversing the cycle of dysfunction may not be easy, it is usually possible. It starts with identifying attainable activities that can lead to physical and psychological re-conditioning that, with gradual increases in activity over time, reverses the collateral losses associated with pain.

## Managing Breakthrough Pain

Chronic pain patients on a steady dose of an opioid pain medication frequently experience episodes of pain that "break through" the analgesic effects of the steady-state drug (whatever the route of administration). Patients and providers therefore need to be prepared, both with knowledge and appropriate analgesics to deal with such breakthrough pain.

Close monitoring by patients of breakthrough episodes is a key step in this process, and providing patients with either paper or electronic pain diaries can greatly facilitate an analysis of the episodes so that correlations can be spotted between the episodes and variables in the patient's life, such as increased or decreased physical activity, use of other substances or medications, changes in disease states, mental-health status, and stress levels. Identifying triggers for breakthrough pain may allow opportunities for making changes that will obviate the need for even more pain medications.

Often, however, a clear causal factor for breakthrough pain is not obvious, and thus, provision should be made to allow patients to deal effectively with that pain without having to resort to visits to emergency rooms or late-night trips to pharmacies.

Therapeutic options for breakthrough pain are not limited to additional opioids—in fact, every effort should be made to find non-opioid methods of dealing with breakthrough pain, i.e., the use of cold or warmth, massage (if indicated), acupuncture, meditation, or electrical stimulation, to name just a few. Unfortunately, insufficient data exist to guide recommendations regarding optimal treatment strategies or specific opioid preparations for breakthrough pain. Clinicians should weigh carefully the potential benefits versus risks when considering the addition of an as-needed opioid to a treatment regimen. The choice of using an opioid for breakthrough pain must be made after all other more optimal treatments have been tried and all risk management and safety concerns have been addressed. Since short-acting opioid preparations may be more desirable as a drug of misuse, clinicians should be especially mindful to firmly educate patients about the potentials for diversion and misuse, and be sure to counsel them on the kinds of safe-storage and disposal procedures. (See Chapter 8.)

In patients at higher risk for aberrant drug-related behaviors or misuse, trial of an as-needed opioid must be weighed against the serious potential for harm. If, after thoughtful consideration of risks and benefits the clinician's medical judgment supports such use, short-acting opioids should only be used in conjunction with substantially heightened monitoring and follow-up. As noted previously, such heightened risk management requires expert consultation and resources that are usually not available in the average clinical setting. As with the management of the underlying chronic pain condition, clinicians should use an agreed-upon set of functional goals as a way to monitor, and if necessary, made adjustments to, the use of as-needed opioid medications. Functional improvements (even if relatively minor) should always be seen—and documented—in order to justify continued prescriptions of medications for breakthrough pain.

## Monitoring Adherence

Monitoring adherence to medication regimens is an imperfect science, but it remains an essential component of periodic review. There are, at present, multiple ways to assess adherence but no single "best" approach. The simplest approach is to just ask patients if they have been taking their medications as prescribed and whether they are achieving their agreed-upon goals. Other methods include pain diaries, written agreements, tablet counts, and laboratory testing. There is no foolproof approach. Effective adherence monitoring usually involves combining several of these techniques.

These methods have both advantages and potential drawbacks. For instance, gross tablet counts are often unreliable because tablets may be discarded, or in the case of opioids, hoarded or diverted and can present inaccurate information about the pattern of medication use. In addition, containers can be lost or intentionally withheld. Patient diaries are questionable representations of reality, particularly when reflecting use of opioids or any other potentially abusable or psychoactive drug. They also may have the undesirable effect of keeping patients dysfunctionally "tuned in" to their pain, rather than allowing them to "get on with their lives." Patient interviews, however, are subject to favorable recall bias on the part of the patient, as well as forgetfulness, especially when the interval between drug use and interview exceeds two weeks.

## Urine Toxicology

Laboratory drug testing remains a widely used part of assessing adherence to a treatment regimen involving controlled substances. Although this type of testing is often expected by regulators and can be used to support optimal care, these tests remain controversial. Some critics of the "trust but verify" approach to pain management cite the lack of clinical evidence that this approach offers more benefits than risks. If, for instance, testing is required only of those suspected of abuse—rather than being required of all patients on chronic opioids as a universal precaution—it can undermine the level of trust between the patient and provider. Even with universal application, some argue the use of such tests undermines trust. Each clinician must determine whether or how such testing should be used. If this testing is employed, as in all therapeutic decisions, it must be used solely in the service of the patient's best interests. Informed consent is an essential element of using urine toxicology screening. This requires patients to understand why the test is used, how it will be interpreted, and how the results of the testing might affect their care.[34, 35]

Urine toxicology tests can be compromised by variability and limitations in obtaining specimens, custody of specimens, laboratory methodologies, and interpreting laboratory data. Effective use of laboratory methodologies requires understanding many details of physiology, pharmacology, and toxicology, which are topics beyond the scope of this discussion. Laboratories vary in their testing methodologies, thresholds, and standards. Results from drug screens may involve diverse drug classes and interpreting them requires clinical understanding well beyond opioids. Clinicians must, therefore, understand these details if toxicology screening is to be used effectively.

Variability may result from differences between laboratories. Some labs, for example, only report values above a certain preset threshold. So, a patient might have a measurable level of a drug, but since it does not exceed the given threshold, it is reported as a "negative" finding. This might lead the clinician to suspect that a prescribed drug, which should be present at the time of drug testing, is absent. The clinician might suspect diversion when, in fact, the drug is being taken properly by the patient. A problem that can arise on the other end of the spectrum is when an abuser who is diverting an opioid attempts to appear compliant with a given medication by taking it only prior to a scheduled or anticipated urine toxicology screen—a practice known as "white coat compliance."

The presence and level of drugs can be detected in serum, urine, hair, and saliva. For routine drug surveillance, urine screening is most commonly used even though such screens are seldom quantitative (i.e., they usually simply confirm the presence or absence of a drug). Serum determination offers quantitative data but is usually not necessary or cost effective in most clinical situations. Testing of serum levels of opioid analgesics in clinical practice is rarely justified, based on the wide variation among patients in minimum effective analgesic concentration, the possible development of tolerance to analgesic or other opioid effects, and considerable variability within any given patient of pharmacokinetic and pharmacodynamic effects. Many comprehensive laboratories are expanding their urine toxicology services and limiting serum analysis to special needs.

Urine is the standard, and often exclusive, specimen used in most laboratory screening for routine drug surveillance of opioids or other controlled substances. Advantages of urine testing include:
- Relative ease of sample acquisition;
- Availability of rapid, inexpensive, and simple testing methods; and
- Longer period of detectability of the drug compared to serum.

Urine screening for opioids is not perfect and generally is one of two types: a screening method or a confirmatory test. (See Table 6.) Specimens found to be negative by the screening method may or may not require confirmation. Clinicians must know the sensitivity and specificity of screening tests for controlled substances. Many point-of-care screens for opiates do not reliably detect opioids other than codeine and morphine, or may not report if levels are below a certain threshold. Therefore, they may give false-negative results for semi-synthetic and synthetic opioid analgesics. Positive samples also may need further study by a confirmatory test.

Another potential source of error in urine opioid testing is consumption by the patient of poppy seeds. Poppy seeds can contain up to

**TABLE 6. SCREENING TESTS**

| | Screening (point of care testing is usually only screening) | Confirmatory |
|---|---|---|
| Analysis Technique | Immunoassay | Gas Chromatography-Mass Spectrometry (GC-MS) or High Performance Liquid Chromatography (HPLC) |
| Sensitivity (power to detect a class of drugs) | Low or none when testing for semi-synthetic or synthetic opioids | High |
| Specificity (power to detect an individual drug) | Varies based on assay used. Can result in false positives and false negatives. | High |
| Use | Qualitative analysis; detects *classes of drugs.* | Quantitative analysis; identifies a specific drug. |
| Cost | Inexpensive (FDA five-drug testing kit ~$1.00) | More expensive, may not be paid for my insurance. |
| Turnaround | On-site, rapid | Slow |
| Other | Intended for use in drug-free population; may not be useful in pain medicine context | Legally defensible results |

This information was provided by Clinical Tools, Inc., and is copyrighted by Clinical Tools, Inc. Adapted from: Opioid Risk.com Appropriate Use of Urine Drug Testing to Improve Patient Care. Available at: http://www.opioidriskcom/print/book/export/html/487. Accessed January 12, 2012.

several hundred micrograms of morphine per gram and up to approximately 50 micrograms of codeine per gram. Concentrations in urine peak within 3 to 8 hours but can linger up to 50 hours after ingestion, hence it is probably best to advise patients undergoing regular or random drug screenings to avoid poppy seeds.

Confirmatory studies are necessary when the consequences of a false-positive or false-negative result are significant, or when identification of specific opioid agents and metabolites is required, such as morphine, oxycodone, and codeine, rather than a class-specific opiate-positive finding. In such cases, it is advisable to use a laboratory that complies with SAMHSA standards, and to use accepted chain of custody procedures for obtaining and handling specimens. (SAMHSA standards are available at: www.workplace.samhsa.gov/)

In the context of family practice settings, unobserved urine collection is usually acceptable. Prescribers, however, should also be aware of the many ways that urine specimens can be adulterated in order to avoid accurate screening. Specimens should be shaken to determine if soap products have been added, for example. The urine color should be noted on any documentation that accompanies the specimen for evaluation since unusually colored urine could indicate adulteration. If possible, urine temperature and pH should be measured. The temperature should be between 32 and 38 °C initially, and can remain warmer than 33 °C for up to 15 minutes. The pH for normal urine can be between 4.5 and 8.

One way to reduce the risk of false positives or false negatives is to develop a relationship with a single laboratory, become familiar with its screening tools and threshold values, and use the same screening tests regularly to build your familiarity with the range of normal results. (For more detailed information about urine drug screening there is a guide for clinicians available at: http://www.mayoclinicproceedings.com/content/83/1/66.full.)

Prescribers also need to be familiar with the metabolites associated with each opioid that may be detected in urine. For instance, a patient who is prescribed codeine might be thought to be using unsanctioned dosages of morphine unless the clinician knows that morphine is a commonly found metabolite of codeine. The same may be true for patients prescribed hydrocodone who appear positive for hydromorphone or oxycodone and oxymorphone. (See Table 7.) Obviously, accusing a patient of non-compliance on the basis of misinterpreted screening data could have significant negative impact on the patient.

**TABLE 7: URINARY ANALYTES OF COMMON OPIOID PAIN MEDICATIONS**

| Drug | Urinary Analytes |
|------|------------------|
| Morphine | Morphine |
|  | Hydromophone |
|  | Codeine |
| Codeine | Codeine |
|  | Morphine |
|  | Hydrocodone |
| Hydrocodone | Hydrocodone |
|  | Hydromorphone |
|  | 6-Hydrocodol |
| Oxycodone | Oxcodone |
|  | Oxymorphone |
|  | Hydrocodone |

Source: Webster LR, and Dove B. Avoiding Opioid Abuse While Managing Pain. Lifesource. 2007.

## Using Prescription Drug Monitoring Programs (PDMPs)

As reviewed in chapters 2 and 10, Prescription Drug Monitoring Programs (PDMPs) can serve an important clinical monitoring role. By using secure internet sites that offer point-of-care access to records of controlled substances from other prescribers and dispensing pharmacies, clinicians can quickly glean patterns of prescription drug use. These patterns may range from verifying the expected treatment course to suggesting multiple prescribing episodes that include numerous prescribers or pharmacies. Currently, each state has a different program with limited sharing between bordering states, although coordination may improve in the future. Some state PDMPs are more comprehensive and accurate than others. (See Chapter 10 for an expanded discussion of this important area.)

## Preventing and Managing Opioid-Related Side Effects

Many patients treated with an opioid will experience some kind of adverse effect. Opioid abuse and addiction are severe adverse events; exactly how often they occur is not known. Constipation is the most common side effect but other possible effects include:

- Sedation
- Urinary hesitancy or retention
- Dry mouth
- Nausea/vomiting
- Itching
- Sweating
- Hypogonadism
- Respiratory depression
- Myoclonus
- Impaired ability to drive

Some side effects, such as sedation, may lessen within a week or two of initiation of treatment. Others, such as constipation, rarely if ever, become less problematic. Constipation is so common, in fact, that when patients use opioids and do *not* have constipation, clinicians should consider possible reasons ranging from rapid bowel transit time to diversion. Constipation requires anticipation, treatment with stimulating laxatives at the time of initiating opioids, and frequent re-evaluation. With the exception of constipation, uncomfortable or unpleasant side effects may potentially be reduced by switching to another opioid or route of administration. (See Appendix F for a chart of treatment options for specific side effects.) Prescribers must remain vigilant to the potential for impaired driving and continually watch for changes that may increase this possibility. The potential for opioids to induce arrythmia is a growing concern related to methadone (discussed in Chapter 7), and may be a concern associated with other opioids.

## Screening for Endocrine Function

Both male and female patients on long-term opioid therapy are at risk for hypogonadism, thus testing endocrine function of all patients should be considered at the start of treatment and possibly annually thereafter. The symptoms of hypogonadism in both genders may include fatigue, mood changes, decreased libido, loss of muscle mass, and osteoporosis.

Table 8 summarizes serum tests that are recommended for both initial assessment and ongoing monitoring of endocrine function.

**TABLE 8. RECOMMENDED ENDOCRINE LAB TESTS FOR PATIENTS ON LONG-TERM OPIOID THERAPY**

| Men | Women |
| --- | --- |
| Total testosterone | Total testosterone |
| Free testosterone | Free testosterone |
| Sex hormone binding globulin | Sex hormone binding globulin |
| Follicle-stimulating hormone | Follicle-stimulating hormone |
| Prolactin | Prolactin |
| | Luteinizing hormone |
| | Dehydroepiandrosterone sulfate |
| | Pregnancy test for premenopausal women not on oral or transdermal contraceptives and who are not having menstrual cycles |

Source: Katz N, and Mazer NA. The impact of opioids on the endocrine system. *Clinical Journal of Pain.* 2009; 25(2):170-5.

## Opioid Rotation

"Opioid rotation" means switching from one opioid to another in order to better balance analgesia and side effects. Rotation may be needed because of a lack of efficacy (often related to tolerance), bothersome or unacceptable side effects, increased dosing that exceeds the recommended limits of the current opioid (e.g., because of co-compounded acetaminophen), or inability to absorb the medication in its present form (i.e., if there is a change in the patient's ability to swallow, switch to a formulation that can be absorbed by a different route such as transdermal.) Nonetheless, there is not substantial evidence showing that opioid rotation is effective or on how to do it most effectively.

Because of the large number of variables involved in how any given opioid will affect any given patient, opioid rotation must be approached cautiously, particularly when converting from an immediate-release formulation to an ER/LA product. An equianalgesic chart should be used when changing from one opioid to another or from one route of administration to another. Such charts must be used carefully, however, since the doses listed are just estimates and can vary. The optimal dose for a specific patient must be determined by careful titration and appropriate monitoring, and clinicians must be mindful that patients may exhibit incomplete cross-tolerance to different types of opioids because of differences in the receptors or receptor sub-types to which different opioids bind. In some cases, because of the risk of potential harm during the time of rotating from one chronic opioid regimen to another, it may be wise to initially use lower doses of the new LA or sustained-release opioid than might be suggested by equianalgesic charts, while temporarily liberalizing, as needed, the use of a short-acting opioid. This would then be followed by gradual titration of the LA opioid to the point where the as-needed short-acting opioid is incrementally reduced, until no longer necessary.

## Managing Non-Adherent Patients

Suspicion that a patient is non-adherent should prompt a thorough investigation, but not a summary rush to judgment. When managing challenging cases and difficult patient-provider relationships, the problem is not always just with the patient. The way clinicians interact with these patients can affect the relationship for better or worse and influence treatment outcomes. The difficult patient may raise a host of reactions in the clinician. Recognizing and managing these reactions is critically important to delivering the best possible care. A clinician's negative reactions to non-adherence might include anger at the patient, disappointment and sadness at the apparent betrayal of trust, or fear that the patient's behavior could expose the provider to legal jeopardy. Scolding, shaming, intimidating, or summarily "firing" a patient are counterproductive—if understandable—responses that may exacerbate, rather than reduce, non-adherent behavior.

It's also important for clinicians to be aware of the distinction between pseudo-addiction and addiction. Patients who are receiving an inadequate dose of opioid medication often "seek" more pain medications to obtain pain relief and may appear compulsive or even dysfunctional. This is called pseudo-addiction, because the behavior is in the service of obtaining a medication that will reduce pain and improve function. Healthcare providers, however, may mistake this for the drug-seeking behavior of true addiction. (Recall that addiction manifests when a person loses control over the use of a substance, uses it compulsively, and continues to use it despite harm and dysfunction.) Some common signs of pseudo-addiction include the following:

- Requesting analgesics by name
- Demanding or manipulative behavior
- Clock watching
- Taking opioid drugs for an extended period
- Obtaining opioid drugs from more than one physician
- Hoarding opioids

Note that these same behavioral signs may also be seen in cases involving addiction. One way to discriminate between the two is to observe as closely as possible the functional consequences of opioid use. (See Table 2 in Chapter 2.) Unlike with addiction, with pseudo-addiction function should improve when the patient obtains adequate analgesia. It remains unclear how often pseudo-addiction occurs. Only with great caution should pseudo-addiction be used as a rationale for continued opioid prescribing, despite a lack of efficacy.

Consultation with an addiction medicine specialist or psychiatrist may be necessary if addiction is suspected or if a patient's behavior becomes so problematic that it jeopardizes a healthy clinician/patient relationship. As always, ambiguous patient behaviors require both vigilance and tempered judgment on the part of the treating clinician.

It can be tempting to assume that patients with chronic pain and a history of non-medical drug use who are not adherent to a treatment regimen are misusing medications. But other causes of non-adherence, such as those discussed above, must be considered before a judgment is reached. If for any reason a clinician's suspicions are aroused, he or she has an obligation to increase vigilance through closer observation, increased testing, and greater involvement of consultants or other supportive clinicians. This vigilant approach to patient monitoring is no different than the management of any patient in whom you suspect toxicity from a drug therapy. Use of patient–provider agreements and/or informed consent documents can guide the steps in this process, and may make implementation more predictable, and hopefully, non-confrontational.

## Components of Effective Monitoring

Clinicians must find the best personal style, work flow and supporting structure that leads to thorough and effective follow up. For many, a structured approach that is applied uniformly across patient groups helps meet the challenge of monitoring each patient on long-term opioid therapy. Several instruments exist that can help with this process. The *Pain Assessment and Documentation Tool* (PADT) is designed to take only a few minutes to collect data on pain relief, activity level, and adverse effects of medications, including potential drug abuse related behaviors. (See Appendix D.) The *Current Opioid Misuse Measure* (COMM) is a relatively simple self-assessment tool that asks patients to describe how they are currently using their medication. (See Appendix D.) No one tool is complete or can provide a single, comprehensive solution.

A patient's progress toward treatment goals may not always be smooth. Reversals and patient frustration are all too common. Clinicians should try to see the long view so that they can better help their patients understand and cope with their condition, or help troubleshoot problems. Here are some tips for effective patient monitoring:

- Listen carefully and compassionately.
- Attend to the entire patient, not just to the pain.
- Refer to relevant health professionals, as needed, to support a treatment plan (e.g., other medical specialists, mental-health professionals, physical therapists, social workers, support groups)
- Adjust pain medications (if indicated and reasonable in the larger context of the patient's situation), and link any adjustments to evidence of improved or decreased function or side effects.
- Modify functional goals as needed. Goals can be expanded with progress, or scaled back if progress is lacking.
- Collaborate with the patient to revise the treatment agreement as needed to reflect changes in treatment regimen, functional goals, or other aspects of the patient's condition.

- In order to make all risks associated with a treatment plan transparent, completely document:
  - All treatment decisions and treatment plan changes, including the risks of *not* taking such actions
  - The ongoing risk management strategy

## Managing Treatment Discontinuation

As mentioned in Chapter 3, treatment plans should include a section on potential discontinuation in cases where the opioid is no longer needed or beneficial or when it has become intolerable or harmful. Reasons for discontinuation can include the healing of or recovery from an injury, medical procedure, or condition; intolerable side effects; lack of response; or discovery of misuse of medications. In cases that do not involve misuse, the goal is to minimize unpleasant or dangerous withdrawal symptoms by tapering the opioid medication slowly, or by carefully changing to a new formulation. Approaches to weaning range from a slow 10% reduction per week to a more aggressive 25 to 50% reduction every few days. In general, a slower taper will produce fewer unpleasant symptoms of withdrawal.

In the case of clear evidence of misuse, treatment must be carefully re-evaluated. Discontinuing an opioid as a result of determining that the risk of therapy outweighs the benefits is always appropriate. A clinician may choose to continue opioid treatment with intensified monitoring, counseling, and careful documentation if it is deemed in the best interest of the patient. However, this requires careful consideration and a well- documented risk management plan that addresses the heightened resources necessary for opioid continuation following evidence of misuse. It must be recognized that the level of vigilance needed for safe continuation often exceeds the abilities and resources of the average prescriber. And if the resources for safe treatment are not available, continuation of treatment is rarely justified.

Discontinuing opioids is not equivalent to discontinuing pain treatment. Evidence that patients have misused an opioid should never be used as the sole justification for terminating them from a practice. Although some patients may no longer benefit from opioids, unless their pain has resolved, other pain treatments are likely to be safer and more effective and should be considered.

If termination of the provider/patient relationship is deemed necessary, clinicians must take care to provide proper transfer of care to

**KEY ELEMENTS OF PERIODIC REVIEW AND FOLLOW-UP***

Relevant history

Outcomes
- Pain assessment
- Assessment of function (compared with previous goals and assessments)

Medication review
- Benefits and adverse effects

PDMP data review (if available)

Examination
- Relevant physical examination
- Mental-health assessment with attention to abuse, addiction and diversion

Laboratory testing
- Urine drug screens (if the clinician deems warranted)
- Other lab tests including endocrine screens

Action plan
- Revise outcomes (ranging from continuing course to major change)

Clarify understandings and expectations

* Note: other elements may be necessary, depending on the individual case.

another provider and ensure that the patient has adequate medications to avoid unnecessary risk, such as from uncontrolled or potentially dangerous withdrawal. Practitioners can be held accountable for patient abandonment if medical care is discontinued without justification or adequate provision for subsequent care. The ethics manual of the American College of Physicians states that "Physician-initiated discontinuation is a serious event, especially if the patient is acutely ill, and should be undertaken only after genuine attempts are made to understand and resolve differences." This same degree of seriousness, sensitivity, and corresponding responsibility on the part of the clinician applies with particular force for patients on opioid therapy for chronic pain.

## Summary

This chapter has reviewed a range of management strategies for patients prescribed opioid therapy for chronic noncancer pain. In the best interest of the patient, prescribers must closely attend to expected treatment outcomes and be alert to a wide range of potential adverse effects. Monitoring a patient's progress toward functional goals requires a partnership between patient and clinician that focuses on the patient's needs as well as a patient who takes charge of attaining treatment goals. The purposes of monitoring and of confirming treatment goals are (1) to help direct and motivate the patient, and (2) to help the clinician determine if treatment is working or is problematic for a variety of reasons. Sometimes functional goals must be calibrated in order to advance treatment outcomes. In the course of periodic review, suspicion that a patient is non-adherent should prompt a thorough investigation of a wide variety of potential underlying causes, but not a summary rush to judgment. In cases that require discontinuation of therapy or discontinuation of the provider/patient relationship, care must be taken to avoid patient abandonment and to continue care (with adequate opioid medications) to minimize unnecessary risk and to maximize the chances that the patient can make progress in another clinical venue.

# Chapter 7
## *Methadone: An Analgesic With Special Risk Factors*

Methadone has recently received growing attention and concern because it is frequently involved in unintentional overdose deaths. These deaths have escalated as methadone has increasingly been used as an analgesic drug for chronic pain. For many years, methadone had been used primarily in specially licensed treatment programs (methadone clinics) for opioid addiction. Its relatively long plasma elimination half-life compared to its relatively short analgesic half-life makes it optimal for maintenance, allowing for once-daily dosing. (A special license is required for clinicians to use methadone and/or buprenorphine in maintenance treatment, but not for using these agents in the treatment of pain.) But methadone also exerts potent analgesic effects in the early phase of its elimination half-life, and this, along with the fact that it is among the least expensive opioids, and has been known to help patients in which other opioids have been unsuccessful, have led to a dramatic increase in its use for alleviating chronic noncancer pain.[28] (When administered by its typical route of delivery—orally or, less commonly, intravenously—methadone is usually given every 4-8 hours. However, methadone also has unique pharmacokinetic and pharmacodynamic characteristics that add substantial risk to its use. For this reason, methadone will be discussed in detail in this chapter.)

Methadone's risk was recently highlighted in a literature review by Webster (2010) of poisoning deaths involving opioids from 1999 to 2009.[36] Although methadone represented less than five percent of all opioids prescribed in this period, it was responsible for a third of the deaths. The major causal factor in this hugely disproportionate risk is believed to be a fundamental misunderstanding on the part of prescribers about the precarious properties of methadone, especially as those properties relate to switching patients to methadone from other opioids. Knowledge about these unique properties of methadone, therefore, is fundamental to its safe and responsible use.

## Pharmacological Properties

Methadone is a synthetic opioid first developed in Germany during World War II and introduced to the United States in 1947. Although its chemical structure is different from classic opioids such as morphine, it acts on the same set of opioid receptors, but does so with different emphasis on the different opioid receptor subtypes. For example, methadone has a lower affinity for the μ-opioid receptor, which some suggest explains why methadone may exert fewer μ-receptor–related side effects such as constipation. However, since methadone use clearly produces significant constipation, this is far from proven. In addition, methadone possess non-opioid receptor effects that may explain some of its potential special efficacy. For instance, it binds to N-methyl D-aspartate (NMDA) receptors, acting as a receptor antagonist to the excitatory neurotransmitter glutamate. Also far from proven, some believe this may be beneficial in reducing opioid tolerance or even hyperalgesia, and may even yield extra efficacy for treating neuropathic pain. It also has monoamine re-uptake inhibition effects. These wide and differential effects across the various opioid receptors, along with its other non-opioid properties, have garnered methadone the reputation of being a "broad spectrum opioid." In light of the recent rise in methadone-related deaths, however, this agent is also building a reputation as an opioid with heightened risk, requiring special prescriber knowledge and patient education for safe use.

Methadone is highly lipid-soluble, which contributes to its very long and highly variable half-life. As illustrated in Figure 5, methadone undergoes a biphasic elimination with a steep early alpha phase (approximately 8-12 hours) followed by a much more gradual beta terminal phase lasting from 30-60 hours.[37] Methadone's analgesic half-life is much shorter than its elimination half-life, which accounts for its different dosing interval for pain compared with addiction maintenance therapy.

This long and variable elimination results from several factors. First, methadone is metabolized by a group of liver enzymes (P450) and other processes that differ from those associated with most other opioids. This predisposes methadone to different drug interactions than would be expected from other opioids. Prescribers who are not aware of this and expect methadone to act like an interchangeable drug with other opioids risk unexpected drug-drug interactions. Also, the liver enzymes that metabolize methadone are subject to significant genetic polymor-

**FIGURE 5: ELIMINATION CURVE FOR METHADONE DEPICTING AN ALPHA PHASE (8-12 HOURS) AND A BETA PHASE (30-60 HOURS)**

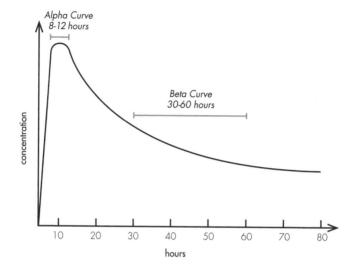

phisms. In some adults, the activity of these enzymes can vary by as much as 50-fold, which contributes to the unpredictability of methadone's effects and side effects. In addition, methadone metabolism can be significantly affected by cigarette smoking (which accelerates elimination) and alcohol consumption (which can augment methadone toxicity acutely and accelerate metabolism with chronic use).

Another potential source of variability in methadone levels comes from methadone's protein-binding properties. Plasma levels of alpha-1-acid-glycoprotein (AAG) can fluctuate widely under the influence of such factors as opioid addiction, cancer, stress reactions, and concurrent administration of drugs such as amitriptyline. High AAG levels may decrease methadone effects and lead to inadequate analgesia or even withdrawal. Alternatively, sudden reduction in AAG levels may increase circulating levels of free/unbound methadone that may transiently expose the individual to greater effects and risk.

For all of these reasons, methadone must be very carefully titrated to avoid overdose. The motto "start low/go slow" is nowhere more apt than in the prescription of methadone!

Recent consensus guidelines from the APS and AAPM recommend a starting dose in most opioid-naive patients of 2.5 mg every 8 hours, with dose increases occurring no more frequently than weekly.[28] The lowest possible dose titration should be followed even in opioid-tolerant patients because methadone appears to be more potent in patients who have been using higher doses of the pre-switch opioid. In older patients or those with renal or hepatic comorbidities, lower starting doses, less frequent dosing, and more cautious dose titration are recommended. Because of its long half-life and variable pharmacokinetics, methadone is not recommended to treat breakthrough pain or as an as-needed medication. In recognition of methadone's long terminal half-life, dose escalation more frequent than 5 half-lives (approximately every 5-7 days) may pose increased risk of accumulation.

## Rotating From Another Opioid to Methadone

Equianalgesic dose ratios for methadone relative to other opioids are variable and can be as little as 1 mg of methadone to every 20 mg of morphine equivalents. In addition, many equianalgesic conversion tables must be used with extreme caution. The consensus recommendations from an expert panel suggest a 75 to 90% *decrement* in the equianalgesic dose from conventional conversion tables when a switch is made from another opioid to methadone.[38]

Clinicians must also guard against assuming that a patient is opioid tolerant based on past prescribed doses. Patients with chronic pain do not always take all of their prescribed medications; hence it is essential to clarify with patients precisely how they have been taking their prescribed medications prior to initiating any change in medications, particularly to methadone. Again, starting low and going slow is best.

An expert panel convened to look into opioid-related deaths concluded that much of the risk for overdose death from methadone results from patients who make mistakes that put them at grave risk.[35] Patients may be driven to misuse opioids by a desire for greater pain relief, to self-medicate a comorbid psychiatric medical condition, or to relieve stress from social, financial, or employment issues related to pain. Because methadone poses greater risks than other opioids, the risk of such behaviors is particularly acute with methadone. Therefore, patients should be educated about these risks and counseled to use methadone exactly as prescribed, and they should be warned about the dangers of mixing unauthorized substances with their medication. Benzodiazepines, in particular, pose a threat. Death investigations often find benzodiazepines have been used in combination with methadone and other opioids. Other respiratory depressants, including alcohol, pose similar risks. Dosing should, therefore, be conservative and cautious until patients demonstrate the ability to tolerate and use the drug safely.

## Cardiac Warnings

On November 27, 2006, the FDA issued a public health advisory warning that methadone can cause serious cardiac conduction disturbances, including QT interval* prolongation and *Torsades de Pointes*, a potentially fatal ventricular arrhythmia.[39] It appears that methadone-related QTc interval prolongation and cardiac arrhythmias can occur at any dose but are more likely at higher doses or with concomitant use of drugs that interact with methadone or that themselves prolong QTc. Although uncommon, the cardiac irregularities that can be induced by methadone can be lethal if not detected. A group from the American College of Physicians has strongly urged clinicians to ask patients about a history of structural heart disease or arrhythmias, and to obtain EKGs before starting methadone, again after 30 days of treatment, and at changes of dosage above 100 mg/day. (See boxed information on page 98 for more details.)[40]

In 2011, SAMHSA convened a multi-disciplinary Expert Panel on the Cardiac Effects of Methadone [*Journal of Addictive Diseases*, 30 (4), 2011]. The Panel suggested that whenever possible, methadone prescribers should have a universal Cardiac Risk Management Plan for all patients, incorporating clinical assessment, personal or family history of structural heart disease, electrocardiogram assessment, risk stratification, and prevention of drug interactions. The panel further endorsed patient-specific risk minimization strategies for patients with identified risk factors for adverse cardiac events, which can include careful patient monitoring, obtaining electrocardiograms as indicated by a particular patient's risk profile, consideration of electrolyte abnormalities, and adjusting the methadone dose as needed—as well as modification of informed consent documents, patient education, and staff education.

---

* QT interval is a measure of the time from the start of the Q wave to the end of the T wave in the heart's electrical cycle. QTc is a corrected QT interval.

---

**RECOMMENDATIONS FOR QTC INTERNAL SCREENING IN METHADONE TREATMENT**

1. Inform patients of arrhythmia risk when prescribing methadone.
2. Ask patients about history of structural heart disease, arrhythmia, and syncope.
3. Obtain pre-treatment electrocardiogram (EKG) for all patients to measure QTc interval, and a follow-up EKG within 30 days (annually thereafter). Additional EKG is recommended if methadone dose exceeds 100 mg/d or if patients have unexplained syncope or seizures.
4. If QTc interval is greater than 450 ms but less than 500 ms, discuss potential risks/benefits with patient and monitor for frequently. If QTc interval exceeds 500 ms, consider discontinuing or reducing the methadone dose, eliminating contributing factors, or using an alternative therapy.
5. Be aware of interactions between methadone and other drugs that possess QT interval-prolonging properties or that slow methadone elimination.

Source: Krantz MJ, et al. QTc interval screening in methadone treatment. *Annals of Internal Medicine*. 2009;150:387-395.

## Potential for Methadone Misuse

Because methadone is used widely to help patients with opioid addiction, some clinicians have the erroneous belief that methadone itself has a lower potential for misuse than other opioids. Although methadone certainly can help patients who misuse heroin and other opioids, it is misused and can be addictive in its own right, both physically and psychologically. In addition, although its withdrawal characteristics are less severe than those of heroin, methadone withdrawal is more prolonged and can be very challenging for patients. Finally, methadone is certainly used illicitly and such use is associated with unintentional overdose deaths, most frequently caused by respiratory depression in the context of simultaneous use with other drugs, such as alcohol or benzodiazepines.

## Methadone Versus Buprenorphine

Buprenorphine is a partial μ-opioid receptor agonist, as opposed to methadone and other commercially available opioids, which are full agonists. Buprenorphine is believed to have less euphoric effects than methadone, which is reflected in the fact that it is classified as a Schedule III drug (methadone is Schedule II). Withdrawal from buprenorphine is also generally less severe than withdrawal from methadone. This, combined with the less-restrictive prescribing associated with buprenorphine, is leading to greater use of this agent in patients on maintenance therapy related to recovery from opioid addiction. (Buprenorphine is also much more expensive than methadone, which limits its use. However, buprenorphine's cost may be mitigated by the increasing availabilty of generic forms.)

Buprenorphine is available in an injectable form, sub-lingual form, and most recently as a transdermal patch. Sublingual buprenorphine is used as a tablet or soluble film for opioid addiction treatment; neither form is approved for the treatment of pain. The patch formulation is FDA approved for chronic pain and is indicated for changing every 7 days. One of the sub-lingual forms includes naloxone, which reduces—though does not eliminate—its potential for misuse. Although buprenorphine has been considered to have reduced misuse potential, it nonetheless clearly is abusable. For example, prison officials in several states have recently reported a rise in attempts to smuggle buprenorphine into prisons by transforming the sublingual product into a paste and spreading it under stamps or over children's artwork.[41] In addition, the thin sub-lingual strips can be easily hidden inside books, magazines, and other items sent to prisoners.

## Summary

Methadone can be an effective analgesic for chronic noncancer pain, but its unique pharmacological characteristics add substantial risk. Deaths involving methadone have increased disproportionately in the past decade, suggesting the need for much greater vigilance on the part of clinicians when prescribing this agent or when switching a patient from another opioid to methadone. Methadone-related deaths have generally occurred in the first two weeks of use due to the initial dose being too high, rapid dose increase, and/or drug interactions. Because of its short analgesic half-life relative to its long terminal half-life, its unpredictable equianalgesic conversion ratios, its variable or unstable metabolism and clearance, its drug interaction profile that differs from other opioids, and its potential cardio-toxicity, methadone use requires advanced knowledge and heightened vigilance and risk management.

# Chapter 8
## Patient Education on Safe Use, Storage, and Disposal of Opioid Medications

*A teenager visits the home of a friend, and while using the bathroom, sees a bottle of hydrocodone on a shelf. Figuring nobody will notice if a few pills are missing, she opens the bottle and pockets a couple of pills.*

*An older adult, wanting to keep his opioid pain medicines handy, keeps the pills in the glove box of his car. His son opens the glove box looking for a map. Seeing the pills and knowing what they are, he waits until his father is out of the car and then takes some of the pills for use later at a party.*

*A college student learns that she is pregnant. She goes to the college health clinic for pre-natal advice, but fails to alert her physician back home, who continues to prescribe extended-release oxycodone for chronic pain related to an old sports injury.*

These stories, drawn from real life, illustrate a critical point: prescribers cannot assume that patients are aware of the many pitfalls associated with having and using opioid medications. Patients require education and guidance. Thorough patient education about such issues as safe use, storage, and disposal of opioid medications is an essential part of responsible opioid prescribing. Patients need to understand that possession and use of opioids is a shared responsibility between the prescriber and the recipient. This responsibility on the part of the patient usually requires both education and the setting of expectations for behavior—and those expectations usually exceed those associated with the use of non-controlled prescription drugs. Just as clinicians have had to adjust to new paradigms of responsible opioid prescribing, patients must adopt a heightened standard of responsible opioid use.

Education about safe use, storage, and disposal should be part of every provider-patient agreement involving opioids. This education can be integrated into standard agreements or informed consent documents. Preparing in advance will help prescribers serve their patients efficiently with minimal interruption of workflow. Meeting this need can take many forms but must offer patient-friendly information at a level that can be widely understood. (Language should be at a sixth- to seventh-grade level or below.)[30, 31] Content may include verbal instructions delivered by a prescriber, nurse or other trained clinic staff person, written handouts, guidance through other media (such as, compact disc—CD, digital versatile disc—DVD, or the Internet), or referral to other resources (such as, a local clinic webpage or national resources). Examples of authoritative patient education can be found at websites, such as PainSafe (www.painsafe.org), the American Pain Foundation (www.painfoundation.org), the National Institutes for Health (NIH)-NIDA Opioid-Risk site (www.opioidrisk.org), and Opioids911-Safety (www.opioids911.org).

## Proper Use

Proper use of opioid medications means that patients carefully follow instructions for use, including special directions about timing of doses, whether to administer the medication with food or without, and any foods or other medications to avoid while administering.[42] Clinicians should be mindful of any physical conditions a patient might have that could interfere with accurate and timely administration of prescribed opioids. For example, patients with low or impaired vision should be advised to wear their glasses when taking their medication and not to take any medication in the dark. Here are some other key ideas to convey to patients about proper use:

- Read the prescription container label each time to check dosage.
- Never use medicines after expiration date.
- Never share medicines with others.
- Do not take a pain medicine with alcohol or other sedatives.
- Do not take a pain medicine to promote sleep.
- Never break, chew, or crush medicines, particularly ER/LA opioid medications.
- For transdermal products, external heat, fever, and exertion can increase absorption, leading to a potentially fatal overdose. In addition, transdermal products with metal foil backings are not safe for use in MRI scanners.

If appropriate and possible, clinicians should also educate caregivers or family members living with the patient to watch for any signs of sedation or impaired breathing, and they should emphasize the fact that respiratory depression is the most serious potential adverse effect of opioids.

Patients should be continually reminded that sharing, selling, or giving away opioids is against the law and poses significant hazards not just to the recipient of the medications, but to society at large. Finally, patients should be encouraged to report any adverse reactions they may experience not only to their physician, but directly to the FDA via the telephone hot line (1-800-332-1088), or the Internet: http://www.fda.gov/safety.

## Dealing With Opioid Overdose

Because respiratory depression is the most serious potential harm from opioids, it is incumbent on clinicians to fully inform patients of this fact and to educate them, their families, and caregivers on recommended steps to take in an emergency. Point out that respiratory depression typically takes some time to develop, hence there will be warning signs of overmedication including:

- Intoxicated behavior—confusion, slurred speech, stumbling;
- Feeling dizzy or faint;
- Acting very drowsy or groggy;
- Unusual snoring, gasping, or snorting during sleep; and
- Difficulty waking up from sleep or of staying awake.

Patients and their caregivers should be counseled to immediately call 911 or an emergency service if they observe any of the following symptoms:

- Person cannot be arouse or wakened, or is unable to talk if awakened;
- Shortness of breath, slow or light breathing, or stopped breathing;
- Gurgling noises coming from mouth or throat;
- Body is limp, seems lifeless;
- Face is pale, clammy;
- Fingernails or lips turning blue/purple; and
- Slow or unusual heartbeat or stopped heartbeat.

If naloxone has been provided to the patient, it should be administered immediately, which will reverse respiratory depression and should allow the patient to begin breathing more normally. (For more information, see Chapter 5.) Given the short half life of naloxone and the possibility that respiratory depression could resume after treatment with naloxone, 911 should be called even if the person appears to have responded to the naloxone administration. If a person has stopped breathing, artificial respiration/cardiopulmonary resuscitation (CPR) should be begun immediately until emergency help arrives. (For more information about steps to take in the event of an overdose, see Opioids911-Safety at www.opioids911.org)

## Safe Storage

Physicians must also educate patients about the importance of proper storage of opioid medicines. This may involve the somewhat delicate suggestion that even children or close relatives can be tempted to use pain medications they have not been prescribed. One way to broach the subject is to refer to recent news stories about, for example, teenagers who obtain prescription medications by taking them from medicine cabinets found in their friends' homes. Some clinicians may choose to have reprints of these news stories available for their patients.

It is best if prescription pain medications (and all controlled substances) are stored in a locked cabinet or other secure storage unit. Storage areas should be cool, dry, and out of direct sunlight. Since bathrooms are often humid and warm, medicine cabinets are not, iron-

---

**SECURE STORAGE**

Controlled substances should be thought of like other valuables in the home, such as jewelry or cash. Patients should be advised to take prescription opioids or other controlled substances out of the medicine cabinet and put them in a secure, but still handy, location. Here are some ideas to suggest:

- An existing safe
- A cut-proof bag designed for travel
- Portable lock boxes designed for travel
- Locking medicine box

ically, often the best place to keep prescription pain medications (medicine cabinets are also seldom lockable). Remind patients not to store medications in their car, to keep medications in the original containers, and to avoid storing medications in the refrigerator or freezer unless specifically directed to do so by a healthcare provider or pharmacist.

Patients, family members, or care-givers should monitor pill containers so they will know if any are pills are missing. Patients often need to be reminded to pay attention to how many pills have been prescribed and how many are used each day. Charting on a daily basis can be very helpful. Innocent errors do occur and early awareness and recognition of the causes, for example, of a patient running out of medication early or needing to refill medication more often than expected, can go a long way toward avoiding false assumptions and unnecessary suspicion.

## Proper Disposal

Proper disposal of unused medications is just as important as proper storage. The Office of National Drug Control Policy currently recommends that unused opioid pain medications be flushed down a toilet. (See Appendix G for the current list of medications recommended by the FDA to be disposed of by flushing.)[43] Some states and municipalities, however, may have different or more stringent guidelines. California, for example, instructs consumers not to flush any medicines down the toilet or drain. If flushing medicines is not allowed in your state, instruct patients to follow the instructions of a pharmacist for disposal or to mix the medicines with an undesirable substance, such as used coffee grounds, put the mixture into a disposable container with a lid or a sealable bag, and place it in the trash.

Here are some other suggestions for educating patients and caregivers about proper disposal of opioid pain medications:

- Conceal or remove any personal information, including the prescription number, on empty containers.
- Explore the availability of drug take-back programs available in the local community and take advantage of these events if possible. The DEA sponsors the National Take Back Initiative which coordinates periodic take-back programs at thousands of state and local law enforcement agencies across the country. More information about these programs can be found at: http://www.deadiversion.usdoj.gov/drug_disposal/takeback/index.html.

## Take-Home Naloxone

As mentioned in Chapter 5, in the future it may become more common to provide patients with intranasal naloxone as a way to reduce the complications associated with accidental overdose. If this is the case, patients will require education about proper administration, storage, and disposal of this opioid antagonist medication as well.

## Pregnancy

For obvious reasons, randomized, controlled clinical trials of the effects of maternal opioid use on fetal development and/or subsequent childhood development have not been conducted. The lack of high-quality studies makes it difficult to evaluate the benefits and risks of opioid medication use by pregnant women (though there has been a significant amount of observation and research with pregnant women in methadone maintenance treatment programs and their newborn children.)

Observational and/or survey data have shown an association between the use of long-term opioid therapy during pregnancy with a range of adverse newborn outcomes, including low birth weight, premature birth, hypoxic-ischemic brain injury, neonatal abstinence syndrome, and neonatal death, though a range of co-related maternal factors may play a role in these associations and causality is not certain. Higher doses of antenatal methadone in tolerant mothers do not seem to increase complication rates.

Nonetheless, given the potential risks of opioids during pregnancy, current APS-AAPM guidelines suggest that clinicians should encourage minimal or no use of opioids during pregnancy unless the potential benefits outweigh risks.[28] If opioid medications are prescribed, clinicians should thoroughly counsel pregnant women about the potential risks and benefits, and clinicians should be prepared to anticipate and manage risks to the patient and newborn.

## Driving and Work Safety

Driving while using opioid medications remains a controversial issue. Particularly at the initiation of therapy, or at times of dose escalation, opioid medications may cause sleepiness, clouded thinking, decreased concentration, slower reflexes, or incoordination, all of which may pose a danger to the patient and others when driving or operating other types of machinery. Irrespective of a number of epidemiologic studies that fail to show an association between long-term opioid use and motor vehicle accidents, fatalities, or citations for impaired driving, clinicians must educate patients about this potentially serious risk and remain alert to treatments or changes in a patient's condition that might impair driving. Since at least some of the cognitive and motor-impairing effects of opioids resolve with steady use and a consistent dose, some activities or driving may be allowable at the discretion of the clinician's medical judgment and in the absence of signs of impairment.

Current APS-AAPM guidelines recommend that all patients who are initially prescribed opioid medications, or those who have their dose adjusted upward, be advised not to drive or engage in potentially dangerous work or other activities.[28] There is no consensus on exactly how long they should abstain from driving. Patients should be educated about the increased risk of impairment when starting opioid therapy, when increasing doses, and when taking other drugs or substances (such as, alcohol, benzodiazepines, or even some cold remedies) that may exacerbate cognitive and motor impairment. Clinicians should be aware that certain professions (i.e., school bus drivers and pilots) may be subject to restrictions in the use of opioid medications. Clinicians should check with their state medical society or the FSMB to obtain up-to-date information in this regard.

## Summary

Responsible opioid prescribing requires clinicians to fully educate patients about the many issues related to safe use, storage, and disposal of opioid pain medications. These task are essential and do not need to be overly burdensome if education is anticipated and you are prepared in advance. By taking seriously the educational component of responsible opioid prescribing, you can make a profound difference in the lives of patients, their loved ones, and society as a whole. Moreover, by doing so, you will more fully meet your requirement for attaining treatment agreement and informed consent. The bottom line is that proactively educating patients is simply good medicine.

# Chapter 9
## *Prescription Drug Misuse Among Young People*

The risks of opioid use and abuse are not limited to adults. Children and young adults (i.e., age 25 and younger) are clearly at risk, and there is a great deal that prescribers can do to help mitigate this serious problem. Prescribers must start by recognizing the problem as well as recognizing their prominent position in helping patients and their families respond appropriately to the various challenges presented by the wide availability of illicit drugs. Although young adult patients and their parents bear responsibility for drug-related behaviors, clinicians can play a valuable role in educating them about the risks of drug misuse by providing information in a neutral setting, by creating a confidential "space" in which young adults can talk freely about drug behaviors, and by dispelling myths surrounding the illicit use of prescription medications. Since caregivers usually accompany children and young adults on visits to clinicians, these encounters provide a special opportunity to educate caregivers and build a partnership with them that may be critical as their children mature. The role of healthcare professionals regarding teen substance abuse is to educate both youths and their parents; help prevent misuse; screen, diagnose, treat and youths who are misusing opioids for nonmedical purposes; refer youths for specialty care, or a combination of these.

While illicit drug use in general has declined among youth in the past decade, rates of nonmedical use of prescription and over-the-counter medications remain alarmingly high.[44] In 2009, one in five U.S. high school students had taken a prescription drug that has misuse potential, such as Oxycontin, Percocet, Vicodin, Adderall, Ritalin, or Xanax, without a doctor's prescription.[45]

Prescription medications, including opioids, are widely available to young people. As illustrated in Figure 6, the bulk of prescription medicines used by high school seniors in the past year were either given to them by or bought from friends or relatives. Young adults can be creative

**FIGURE 6. SOURCE OF PRESCRIPTION NARCOTICS OTHER THAN HEROIN AMONG THOSE WHO USED IN THE LAST YEAR (GRADE 12), 2009-2011**

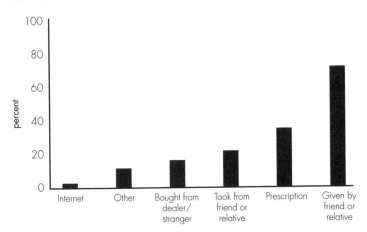

*Numbers do not add up to 100% because some respondents obtained prescription drugs from more than one source.*

Adapted from: Johnston LD, O'Malley PM, Bachman JG, Schulenberg JE. (2010). Monitoring the Future national results on adolescent drug use: Overview of key findings, 2010. Ann Arbor: Institute for Social Research, The University of Michigan.

in finding ways to obtain prescription medications. For example, there are reports of young adults who attend real estate open houses in order to search medicine cabinets for prescription medications. Such medications may be brought to parties and shared indiscriminately with others, with little or no information provided about what the medications are or what effects they might have and what risks non-medical use entail. Some young adults report that prescription medications are sometimes dumped into a bowl or other container (creating what is called "trail mix") and attendees at such "pharming" parties simply take as much as they want. In such situations, the combination of prescription medications with alcohol or cannabis is common and greatly increases the risks of dangerous behaviors, harmful effects, or death.

It is also an unfortunate reality that prescription drugs may be obtained legitimately by young people, but then may be shared with others. As illustrated in Figure 7, the rate of prescription opiate use rises significantly during the teen years.[46]

Relatively easy access to prescription medications is coupled with a broad ignorance about the true nature of these medications among

**FIGURE 7: OPIATE UTILIZATION IN CHARLESTON COUNTY, SC**

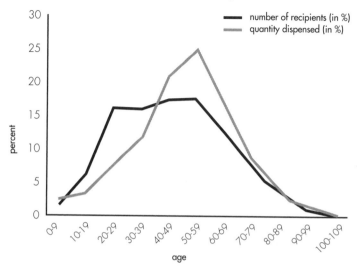

Source: Surgeon General's Expert Panel on Prescription Drug Abuse in Youth: Prescription Monitoring Program Roles. U.S. Department of Health and Human Services, March 29, 2011.

youth. In 2005, for example, the Partnership for a Drug-Free America conducted a study of teen attitudes, which came to the following conclusions:[47]

- 19% of teens reported using prescription medications to get high.
- 40% of teens believe that prescription medications are "much safer" to use than illegal drugs.
- 31% believe there's "nothing wrong" with using prescription medicines without a prescription "once in awhile."
- 29% believe prescription pain relievers are not addictive.

A survey of teen attitudes and knowledge of drugs and alcohol that was released in 2011 found that about 1 in 4 teens knows at least one friend or classmate who uses prescription drugs without a prescription to get high.[48]

Clearly, parents, schools, and healthcare providers must do a better job of educating young people about the risks associated with opioid pain medications and other prescription drugs! Although several groups share this responsibility for mitigating substance misuse, clinicians are powerfully positioned to have a positive impact on young people's attitudes about using prescription medications, for the following reasons:[49]

- The time when a young adult is being seen by a healthcare provider for either a routine checkup or a problem related to substance use is an ideal "teachable moment" when information is more likely to be heard and absorbed.

- Young patients often come to doctor appointments with their parents or other influential relatives or individuals, offering physicians an opportunity to address young patients when they might be most receptive while supported by family or other adults.

- Healthcare providers are often seen as trusted adult figures, and the confidentiality conferred by the physician/patient relationship may help young adults be more open and honest about their misuse of prescription medicines.

- Clinicians can provide anti-substance abuse messages in the neutral context of a general risk to health, rather than in more threatening or accusatory legal, familial, or moral contexts.

When talking to young people or their parents, clinicians should bear in mind the following points:

- Explain the hazards of opioid pain medications without demonizing the medicines or implying that they have no legitimate role in medicine.

- Point out that the medicine cabinets at home and at the homes of friends are extremely easy targets for young people and that even "good" kids can be tempted to experiment, especially in response to peer pressure.

- Use reflective listening approaches. (See Chapter 2.)

- Avoid language or inflection that would suggest you are trying to "be the parent" or, if talking to a parent, that would suggest you are trying to tell parents how to do their job.

- Remind young patients that misusing prescription drugs (not just pain medications) is linked to a wide range of risks including injury, overdose, physical or sexual assaults, teen pregnancy, sexually transmitted diseases (STDs), learning problems, and brain damage.

- Be prepared to provide your patients and their parents or guardians with additional resources including pre-prepared take-home materials and recommended websites.

Both the AMA and the American Academy of Pediatrics recommend that annual screening for substance use be part of routine adolescent care, but primary care physician adherence to these recommendations is low. According to the American Academy of Pediatrics, fewer than 50% of primary care physicians (PCPs) screen all adolescents for substance use, and less than 12.5% screen for such misuse by using a structured tool.[50] Screening for substance use/misuse is recommended as a regular part of adolescent pain management, and employing a structured screening tool may be particularly appropriate.

It is also recommended that young adult patients who seek urgent or emergency medical care be screened for substance use, since urgent care workers may reach youth who already are experiencing consequences of substance use, youth who lack a primary care physician, or both.

Young adults who screen positive for substance use but have not yet developed clinical disorders may be helped by brief interventions using established protocols such as those developed by The National Center on Addiction and Substance Abuse at Columbia University (www.casacolumbia.org). Short counseling sessions using motivational interviewing techniques may help prevent future substance use and can be administered by physicians or other trained staff.

As stressed above and elsewhere, preparation for positive interventions and "teachable moments" is critical to success. Clinicians must not assume that their direct interaction will be sufficient for sustained impact, and must be prepared to provide additional helpful information (such as, printed hand-outs, recommended books, or websites) to parents, guardians, and/or grandparents about the problem of young adult use of prescription medications, as well as suggest approaches to prevention or intervention. It may be helpful, for example, to convey to the parents the following signs that a teenager may be using alcohol, opioids, or other illicit drugs:[51]

- Association with a new group of friends who concern you or who you don't know.
- Slipping grades.
- Loss of interest in hobbies, sports, or other favorite activities.
- Change in eating or sleeping patterns.
- Deterioration of personal grooming or hygiene.
- Hostile, uncooperative behavior.
- Being frequently late for deadlines or curfews.

- Red-rimmed eyes and a runny nose, but no allergies or a cold.
- Disappearing household money, prescription drugs, cough medicine or any other sedating or stimulating medications.

The same principles of responsible opioid prescribing that a clinician uses with adults should be applied when the patient is a child or young adult. All of the steps for proper evaluation, patient education, informed consent, initiation of treatment and the setting of functional treatment goals that have been detailed in previous chapters should be followed when prescribing opioids to young people.

## Summary

Clinicians should remember that the misuse of opioid pain medications is not limited to adults. Significant numbers of young people are currently using these drugs, often with little knowledge of (or even dangerous misconceptions) about their true risks.

Clinicians are well-positioned to have a positive impact on children and their parents because they can provide advice and information in a neutral context and can listen to concerns and questions that a young person might have in a confidential atmosphere. Screening for substance use/misuse should be a regular part of adolescent care, and the use of structured screening tools is recommended. In addition, anyone receiving controlled substances should be educated about the potential for these medications to be misused by children or young adults. Providing education about preventive actions and teaching basic risk management to anyone receiving controlled substances is an integral part of responsible care.

# Chapter 10
## *Legal and Regulatory Issues*

Because of their potential for abuse, opioid medications are controlled substances. Consequently, they and the healthcare professionals who prescribe, administer, or dispense them are regulated by a complex series of federal and state policies on controlled substances, as well as other state laws and regulations that govern healthcare practice. Such policies are intended to prevent drug abuse and substandard prescribing practice. But in some cases, their impact extends beyond their intended purpose in ways that can hamper legitimate medical practices and create barriers for caregivers and patients.

Although considerable progress has been made in the past decade to amend state laws in hopes of striking balanced regulatory policies that offer access to appropriate care for legitimate patients, significant state-to-state inconsistencies remain. Some state policies may create particular practice standards that differ from national conventions. Growing attention to the separate public health crises of under-treated pain and prescription drug abuse are leading to calls for more circumspect and specific regulations. Some state laws have been recently revised or are in the process of revision. Prescribers should be aware of the legal language in their states' professional and business codes. Some of these provisions may include:

- Limits on the amounts of opioids that can be prescribed and dispensed or limits on associated refills or timing for follow-up evaluation.
- Listing opioids as treatments of last resort.
- Requirements that using opioids for chronic pain be associated with documented functional outcomes.
- Requirement for formal evaluation by a "pain specialist" if the patient is using greater than a certain dose of an opioid.
- Requirement that prescribers take a certain number of hours of CME education in pain management or opioid prescribing.

Language that can enhance pain management is being added to some state policies and laws. Exactly how best to address the needs of patients in pain as well as the public's need for safety in dispensing controlled substances, however, is an area of controversy. Several states have sought to redefine their policies, but their impact on reducing prescription drug abuse or under-treated pain is not clear. It is imperative, however, that prescribers are thoroughly familiar with their own state's laws and regulatory practice standards. (Access to these laws, or summaries of the laws, is available through the FSMB website: http://www.fsmb.org/pain-resources.html.)

Unfortunately, evidence suggests that many clinicians remain ignorant of the state regulations under which they practice. This may have problematic consequences: on the one hand, some prescribers may limit their use of controlled substances in the mistaken belief that their state laws are restrictive or overly punitive; on the other hand, some may be practicing in a manner inconsistent with accepted standards and this might be viewed as potentially suspicious by their state's regulatory agencies that oversee medical practice.

Prescribers also must have a firm grasp of the federal laws relating to controlled substances. These laws are articulated in the federal Controlled Substances Act (CSA), which attempts to balance the competing demands of both control and availability. Under this act, licensed professionals can prescribe, dispense, and administer controlled substances for legitimate medical purposes in the course of professional practice. (Note that most opioid analgesics are Schedule II drugs although a few, which happen to be the most prescribed, are schedule III drugs. Schedule I analgesics, such as heroin, are considered to have no legitimate medical uses.) The "control" portion of the CSA attempts to prevent diversion, establishes a system of secure manufacture and distribution, requires record-keeping procedures, and sets up penalties (including criminal prosecution) for violating its provisions.

## Prescription Drug Monitoring Programs (PDMPs)

As noted in Chapter 6, many states and the federal government have promoted prescription drug monitoring programs (PDMPs) as a way to help limit misuse of medications and also provide a tool for healthcare providers to make sound clinical decisions. These PDMPs are not new, though their emergence has been slow. California and Hawaii enacted PDMPs in the 1940s. By the 1980s, seven more states had added PDMPs. These early programs required that physicians use state-issued multiple copy forms (duplicate or triplicate) to write prescriptions for Schedule II controlled substances, and that pharmacies return one copy to the state after dispensing a drug. Physicians were usually required to obtain prescription forms from a state law enforcement agency and some states charged a fee for the forms or limited the number that could be ordered at any time.

As of early 2012, forty states have operational PDMPs and nine others have enacted legislation and programs that are not yet operational. This is a changing regulatory landscape. Updates for each state can be found at http://www.pmpalliance.org/content/state-profiles-reports. Each of these state PDMPs has varying organizational structures and activities. For instance, PDMPs in most states are housed in the state department of health or in the state pharmacy board, whereas some come under the state law enforcement agency, a professional licensing agency, a substance abuse agency, or a consumer protection agency. Moreover, there is variability in the drugs and drug schedules that operational programs monitor (i.e., 22 collect data on Schedule II-V, 16 on II-IV, one on II-III, and one on Schedule II only, while several collect information on non-controlled drugs of concern).* Most programs are now designed for use by clinicians while others remain systems with sole access by law enforcement.

Most states are now moving to computerized PDMPs. In such systems, pharmacies transmit data to the state on controlled substance prescriptions. Historically, federal funding has come from Harold Rogers PDMP Grants administered through the U.S. Department of Justice's Bureau of Justice Assistance. In practice, PDMPs take different forms because each state government is charged with determining the goals, structure, and organization of its program. Variation among states is still common, even in states that border each other and must deal with patients crossing state lines for care. This situation may improve since the federal government has made nationwide prescription monitoring a central pillar of its action plan on prescription drug abuse and has emphasized the need for sharing data across state lines.

Certain characteristics of PDMPs can have a deterrent effect on potential criminal activities. For example, some state authorities report

---

* These state-based programs are alternately called prescription monitoring plans (PMPs) or PDMPs, depending on the state. For clarity, this book refers to all these programs as PDMPs.

that use of tamper-resistant prescription forms significantly reduces or eliminates prescription forgery. Thus, while government-issued serialized prescriptions have largely been abandoned as useful tools for prescription monitoring, the use of security paper that is tamper-resistant is increasing. These security-paper prescription forms employ the same technology that has long been used on personal bank checks or on paper money—these include a watermark that may be viewed at a certain angle, photochromic features that produce an image such as the word "void" if the paper is copied or scanned by a light source, or even thermochromic features in which the paper changes color when touched by warm fingers or a heat source.

Increasingly, PDMPs are making prescribing information available to practitioners at the point of clinical care for the purpose of identifying prescribing trends. These data can help prescribers identify people who are receiving the same opioid from multiple prescribers and/or multiple pharmacies. Such individuals may have perfectly acceptable reasons for these multiple prescribing episodes, but the existence of such a pattern should always trigger inquiry. Further action could range from a simple re-evaluation of the treatment plan to criminal prosecution, depending on the circumstances of the case.

The PDMP as a bedside tool is new to many prescribers and will require time for incorporation into widespread practice. All of the potential benefits of PDMPs are unlikely to be known until we fully integrate user-friendly and accessible systems into the daily clinical practice of all prescribers of controlled substances. Such enhanced systems will require training for clinicians, technological solutions that offer data reliability, security, uniformity, and compatibility across state lines, as well as outcomes research.

Contemporary PDMPs are not intended to interfere with medical practice, and are increasingly being designed to reduce potential barriers to care. Unlike PDMP programs of the past that were intrusive to clinicians and negatively influenced prescribing practices, newer electronic-based PDMPs collect data behind the scenes of clinical care. Likewise, contemporary PDMPs typically do not require prescribers to obtain prior approval to issue prescriptions and they do not impose limits on the quantity that may be prescribed. Limitations on prescribing controlled substances do exist, but are governed by state laws that are separate from those related to PDMPs.

# Federal Guidelines for Prescribing Controlled Substances

In 2006, the DEA released an updated Practitioner's Manual that summarizes and explains the basic requirements for prescribing, administering, and dispensing controlled substances under the CSA. The complete manual is available online (www.deadiversion.usdoj.gov), and prescribers are urged to read it carefully. The DEA website is also worth checking periodically for any updates that may occur. The DEA also issued a clarification of its policies relating to the use of controlled substances for pain that appeared in the September 6, 2006 Federal Register. This document is titled Dispensing Controlled Substances for the Treatment of Pain. Selected passages are posted on www.fsmb.org/pain and clarify the following topics:

- The Statutory Role of DEA in Regulating the Prescribing of Controlled Substances.
- The Meaning of the "Legitimate Medical Purpose" Requirement.
- Other Recurring Questions:
  - What are the potential signs to a clinician that a patient might be seeking drugs for the purpose of abuse or diversion?
  - What are the general legal responsibilities of a prescribers to prevent diversion and abuse when prescribing controlled substances?
  - What additional precautions should be taken when a patient has a history of drug abuse?

In the fall of 2007, the DEA issued a final ruling that amends its regulations to allow practitioners to provide individual patients with multiple prescriptions, to be filled sequentially, for the same schedule II controlled substance. These multiple prescriptions allow a prescriber to write, and a patient to receive, sequential prescriptions for up to a 90-day supply of that controlled substance. Thus practitioners may write multiple prescriptions, each dated the day the prescriptions are written, but only one would be for immediate filling while the others would have sequential and non-overlapping fill dates. The intervals are up to the prescriber so that it might be days, weeks, or months. For instance, a prescriber might state "do not fill until 30 days from prescription date" or "do not fill until 60 days from prescription date," etc. (Details of this ruling are available at www.deadiversion.usdoj.gov/fed_regs/rules/2007/fr1119.htm.)

In 2010, the DEA adopted new rules allowing prescribers who are registered with the DEA to prescribe scheduled substances electronically. The same rules allow pharmacies to receive, dispense, and archive electronic prescriptions. (Details are available at www.deadiversion. usdoj.gov/ecomm/e_rx/.)

## Summary

Current federal regulations, emerging state laws, and practitioner guidelines from professional organizations seek rational strategies for providing patients with safe and effective pain relief. Prescribers who find such balance in their practice will likely find themselves congruent with the goals of regulators, and most important, with the needs of their patients. New or revised regulations, and the reality of changing or inconsistent existing regulations at both federal and state levels, reinforce the fundamental message of this chapter: physicians must take the time to educate themselves about the realities of the legal environment in which they practice and remain up to date on any changes to those policies.

# Conclusion
## *Pharmacovigilance is Good Medicine*

In light of the alarming rise of rates of prescription drug abuse, the use of opioids in the treatment of chronic noncancer pain is increasingly controversial. The Institute of Medicine's estimate that 100 million Americans are in chronic pain, incurring direct and indirect expenses of $635 billion per year, speaks to the dramatic costs and immeasurable suffering associated with chronic pain. Clinicians cannot afford to get this wrong.

The public health crisis of prescription drug abuse confronts clinicians with what may seem like a narrowing window in which to determine appropriate care. On one hand, we are compelled to relieve our patients' suffering and help them regain function in their lives. On the other hand, we must be responsible when prescribing medications that are easily misused or abused. My contention is that the balancing act inherent in responsible opioid prescription is neither unique nor uniquely burdensome for clinicians, and that, ultimately, patients, society, and clinicians are best served by treating pain with a rational approach that safely and effectively includes the judicious use of opioids. Walking this middle path requires that prescribers apply basic principles of safety and efficacy to balance the needs of patients in pain with the need to minimize the potential harms from opioid abuse and diversion. For instance, prescribers of opioids must firmly recognize that opioids may help some patients, but they certainly do not help everyone; and that when a reasonable amount of an opioid does not produce a desired outcome, increasing the dose without factoring the possibility of either diminishing returns or escalating risk is not in the patients' best interests.

Current professional guidelines for prescribing opioids do not provide complete details on using controlled substances for pain management. Nor do they set inflexible standards of medical practice. Rather, they provide a basic framework by which clinicians, medical boards, and other regulators can assess whether practice is within the current standard of care. I believe that this current standard of care offers prescribers ample margin for medical judgment, while it demands increased risk management and use of objective evidence of treatment outcomes. Recommendations on specific drugs, formulations, dosages, duration of treatment, or other variables are seldom provided in professional guidelines because these are details of care that require medical knowledge, information related to individual patients, and reasoned medical judgment. In short, the standard of care now requires an informed and engaged treating clinician.

This book focuses on process-oriented aspects of care and describes a realistic approach to opioid prescribing that can readily be integrated into daily clinical practice. Most of these recommended steps are also appropriate when prescribing drugs that are not controlled, as well as for the use of non-pharmacological treatments. Nonetheless, no practice guidelines can substitute for a prescriber's compassion and commitment.

Despite major efforts to add scientific certainty to the practice of opioid therapy for pain, medical evidence is not robust and a great deal remains to be learned and translated into clinical practice. Although regulators appropriately ask physicians to be as vigilant as possible in managing the risks associated with opioid pain medications, exactly how that vigilance is best deployed is still left to the medical judgment of the clinicians. Accordingly, clinicians must remain alert to new developments in research and drug development, as well as to changes in state or federal regulations.

> *Pain Medicine is a young discipline still vastly under-represented in medical education curricula and residency programs. This glaring deficiency must be reversed.*

I do not believe that the vast majority of clinicians resist treating pain because they lack compassion—but I do believe that the associated legal and regulatory hassles can lead some clinicians to use less-effective agents, or even to avoid treating patients with chronic pain conditions. In addition, many physicians are not well trained or equipped to manage chronic pain. Although pain is the most common reason a patient will seek medical help, pain physiology, and it assessment and treatment, are barely taught to most clinicians in training. This can result in an inadequate knowledge base among clinicians and may also create barriers to the creation of healthcare systems in which chronic pain can be treated most effectively. The delivery of high-quality care for chronic pain crosses traditional disciplines in medicine and challenges many long-held, but scientifically unsupported attitudes of some practitioners. Few clinicians have the privilege of working in a truly state-of-the-science pain clinic that is fully equipped to handle the complex assessment, treatment and follow-up care necessary for all patients in pain. Nonetheless, every clinical practice must be able to treat pain at some level, and every practitioner will be well served by preparing to meet this challenge by implementing systems that support necessary patient education and risk management. New medical information systems reduce the clinician's burden of providing all the patient education, comprehensive informed consent, initial and follow-up assessments, consistent checkup and data comparison, and complete documentation required if one is to follow best practices. But even without having such systems in place, busy clinicians can still implement the steps outlined in this book.

Meanwhile, the science and technology of pain medicine is expanding rapidly with new developments in basic research and new pharmacological and non-pharmacological options that have increased efficacy and reduced risk. Each clinician has a responsibility to achieve and maintain a working understanding of pain management, and if you choose to prescribe opioids or other controlled substances, a solid grounding in safe and effective prescribing practices.

# Abbreviations

| | |
|---|---|
| AAG | alpha-1-acid-glycoprotein |
| AAPM | American Academy of Pain Medicine |
| ADH | antidiuretic hormone |
| AMA | American Medical Association |
| APS | American Pain Society |
| ASSIST | alcohol, smoking, and substance involment screening test |
| CAGE | cut down on drinking or drug use, annoyed or angered by others, felt guilty, eye opener (a screening tool) |
| CD | compact disc |
| CDC | Centers for Disease Control and Prevention |
| CHF | congestive heart failure |
| CME | continuing medical education |
| CNCP | chronic noncancer pain |
| COMM | current opioid misuse measure |
| COPD | chronic obstructive pulmonary disease |
| COT | chronic opioid therapy |
| CSA | Controlled Substances Act |
| DEA | (U.S.) Drug Enforcement Administration |
| DIRE | diagnosis, intractability, risk, efficacy |
| DoD | (U.S.) Department of Defense |
| DSM | Diagnostic and Statistical Manual (of Mental Disorders) |
| DVD | digital versatile disc |
| EKG | electrocardiogram |
| ER | extended release |
| FDA | (U.S.) Food and Drug Administration |
| FSMB | (The) Federation of State Medical Boards (of the United States, Inc.) |
| GC-MS | gas chromatography-mass spectrometry |
| HIV | human immunodeficiency virus |
| HPLC | high performance liquid chromatography |
| IASP | International Association for the Study of Pain |
| LA | long-acting |
| MAOI | monoamine oxidase inhibitor |

| | |
|---|---|
| MRI | magnetic resonance imaging |
| NIDA | National Institute on Drug Abuse |
| NIH | National Institutes of Health |
| NMDA | N-methyl D-aspartate (receptor) |
| NSAIDS | non-steroidal anti-inflammatory drugs |
| ORT | Opioid Risk Tool |
| PADT | pain assessment and documentation tool |
| PCP | primary care physician |
| PDMP | prescription drug monitoring program |
| PDUQ | prescription drug use questionnaire |
| PMQ | pain medication questionnaire |
| QT | QT interval is a measure of the time from the start of the Q wave to the end of the T wave in the heart's electrical cycle |
| QTc | corrected QT interval |
| REMS | risk evaluation and mitigation strategies |
| SAMHSA | Substance Abuse and Mental Health Services Administration |
| SCID | structured clinical interview for DSM disorders |
| SISAP | screening instrument for substance abuse potential |
| SOAPP-R | screener and opioid assessment for patients with pain—revised |
| SODQ | severity of opiate dependence questionnaire |
| STAR | screening tool for addiction risk |
| STD | sexually transmitted disease |
| VA | Veterans Administration |
| VAS | (standard) visual analog scale (for pain) |

# References

1  U.S. Food and Drug Administration (FDA). Blueprint for Prescriber Continuing Education Program. November 4, 2011.

2  Executive Office of the President of the United States. Epidemic: Responding to America's Prescription Drug Abuse Crisis. 2011.

3  Volkow ND. Quote to the U.S. Senate Committee pm Crime and Drugs, Committee on the Judiciary and the Caucus on International Narcotics Control United States Senate. March 12, 2008.

4  Joint meeting of the anesthetic and life support drugs advisory committee and the drug safety and risk management advisory committee. Risk evaluation and mitigation strategies for extended-release and long-acting opioid analgesic. July 22 and 23, 2010.

5  Substance Abuse and Mental Health Services Administration (SAMHSA). Treatment Episode Data Set. Substance Abuse Treatment Admissions Involving Abuse of Pain Relievers. SAMHSA; 1998 and 2008. July 15, 2010.

6  United States Department of Justice, Drug Enforcement Administration (DEA), Office of Diversion Control. Practitioners Manual: An Informational Outline of the Controlled Substances Act. DEA; Washington, DC. 2006. Available at www.deadiversion.usdoj.gov/pubs/manuals/pract/index.html

7  SAMHSA. Trends in emergency department visits involving nonmedical use of narcotic pain relievers. The Drug Abuse Warning Network (DAWN) report. SAMHSA. http://store.samhsa.gov/product /DAWN10-0618. Accessed March 4, 2011.

8  SAMHSA. Substance abuse treatment admissions by primary substance of abuse, according to sex, age group, race, and ethnicity, 2008: treatment episode data set (TEDS). Drug and Alcohol Services Information System. SAMHSA. http://wwwdasis.samhsa.gov/webt/quicklink /US08.htm. Accessed February 25, 2011.

9  Fingerhut LA. Increases in Poisoning and Methadone-Related Deaths: United States, 1999-2005. National Center for Health Statistics (NCHS), Health and Stats. February 2008.

10  Centers for Disease Control and Prevention (CDC). Unintentional drug poisoning in the United States, July 2010. National Center for Injury Prevention and Control, CDC. http://www.cdc.gov/HomeandRecreatonalSafety/pdf/poison-issue-brief.pdf. Accessed March 16, 2011.

11  Institute of Medicine. Relieving Pain in America: A blueprint for transforming prevention, care, education, and research. Report Brief. June 2011.

12  National Institute of Neurological Disorders and Stroke. Low back pain fact sheet. Available from www.ninds.nih.gov/health_and_medical. Accessed January 12, 2012.

13  NCHS. Health, United States, 2006 with Chartbook on Trends in the Health of Americans. Hyattsville, MD: U.S. Department of Health and Human Services; 2006.

14  American Cancer Society (ACS). Cancer Facts and Figures 2012. Atlanta: ACS; 2012.

15  Weiss SC, Emanuel LL, Fairclough DL, Emanuel EJ. Understanding the experience of pain in terminally ill patients. Lancet. 2001; 357:1311-1315.

16 Federation of State Medical Boards (FSMB). Model Policy for the Use of Controlled Substances for the Treatment of Pain. FSMB, Dallas, TX. Available at http://www.fsmb.org/pdf/2004_grpol_Controlled_Substances.pdf. Accessed April 20, 2011.

17 Scarry E. *The Body in Pain*: The Making and Unmaking of the World. Oxford University Press. New York, NY. 1985.

18 Tang NK, Crane C. Suicidality in chronic pain: a review of the prevalence, risk factors, and psychological links. *Psychological Medicine* 2006; 36:575-586.

19 Gourlay D, Heit H. Universal precautions: a matter of mutual trust and responsibility. *Pain Medicine*. 2006; 7(2):210-211.

20 Wu SM, Compton P, Bolus R, et al. The addition behaviors checklist: validation of a new clinician-based measure of inappropriate opioid use in chronic pain. *Journal of Pain and Symptom Management* 2006;32:342-351.

21 U.S. Drug Enforcement Administration (DEA). Supervisory Training: Guidelines for a Drug Free Workplace. 4th ed. Alexandria, VA. DEA; 2003.

22 Alliance of States with Prescription Monitoring Programs. Available at: http://www.pmpalliance.org

23 The PMP Center of Excellence. Available at http://pmpexcellence.org. Accessed January 18, 2012.

24 Bergman v Wing Chin, MD and Eden Medical Center, No. H205732-1 (Cal App Dept Super Ct 1999).

25 Cleeland CS, Ryan KM. Pain assessment: global use of the Brief Pain Inventory. *Annals of the Academy of Medicine*, Singapore. 1994; 23(2):129-138.

26 Payne R, Anderson E, Arnold R, et al. A rose by any other name: pain contracts/agreements. *American Journal of Bioethics*. 2010;10(11):5-12.

27 *American Journal of Bioethics*, All articles in this special issue. December 2010, vol. 10, no. 11.

28 Chou E, Fanciullo GJ, Fine PG, et al. Clinical Guidelines for the Use of Chronic Opioid Therapy in Chronic Noncancer Pain. *The Journal of Pain*. 2009;10(2):113-130.

29 Management of Opioid Therapy for Chronic Pain Working Group. VA/DoD clinical practice guideline for management of opioid therapy for chronic pain. Washington (DC): Department of Veterans Affairs, DoD; May 2010.

30 Roskos SE, Keenum AJ, Newman LM, Wallace LS. Literacy demands and formatting characteristics of opioid contracts in chronic nonmalignant pain management. *Journal of Pain*. 2007;8(10):753-758.

31 Center for Professional Practice of Nursing. Guidelines for preparing patient education handouts. UC Davis Health System. Available at: http://www.ucdmc.ucdavis.edu/cne/health_education/guide.html. Accessed July 22, 2011.

32 Albert S, Brason II F, Sanford CK, et al. Project Lazarus: Community-Based Overdose Prevention in Rural North Carolina. *Pain Medicine*. 2011(Jun);12(Suppl s2):S77-S85.

33 American Medical Association (AMA). The physician's role in medication reconciliation: issues, strategies and safety principles. 2007.

34 Rich BA. Trust But Verify? The ethics of opioid agreements for patients with chronic pain. San Francisco Medical Society website. Available at http://www.sfms.org. Accessed August 29, 2011.

35  Arnold RM, Han PKJ, Seltzer D. Opioid contracts in nonmalignant pain management: objectives and uncertainties. *The American Journal of Medicine.* 2006;119:292-296.

36  Webster LR, et al. Select medical-legal reviews of unintentional overdose deaths. Presented at 26th Annual Meeting of AAPM; February 3-6, 2010: San Antonio, TX.

37  Fishman SM, Wilsey B, Mahajan G, Molina P. Methadone reincarnated: novel clinical applications with related concerns. *Pain Medicine.* 2002;3(4):339-348.

38  Knotkova H, Fine PG, Portenoy RK. Opioid rotation: The science and limitations of the equianalgesic dose table. *Journal of Pain Symptom Management.* 2009;38(3): 426-439.

39  Food and Drug Administration. Public Health Advisory: Methadne Use for Pain Control May Result in Death and Life-Threatening Changes in Breathing and Heart Beat. November 27, 2006.

40  Krantz MJ, Martin J, Stimmel B, Mehta D, Haigney MC. QTc interval screening in methadone treatment. *Ann Intern Med.* 2009;150:387-395.

41  Goodnough A, Zezima K. When Children's Scribbles Hide a Prison Drug. *New York Times.* May 26, 2011.

42  American Pain Foundation. Six Opioid Safety (SOS) Steps: When opioids are prescribed for your pain. 2010.

43  Office of National Drug Control Policy. Proper Disposal of Prescription Drugs. October, 2009. Available at: www.whitehousedrugpolicy.gov. Accessed May 17, 2011.

44  Substance Abuse and Mental Health Services Administration (SAMHSA). Results from the 2009 National Survey on Drug Use and Health: Volume 1. Summary of National Findings. Office of Applied Studies, NSDUH Series H-38A, HHS Publication No. SMA 10-4586Findings. 2010.

45  The Partnership for a Drug-Free America. The Partnership Attitude Tracking Study (PATS) Teens in grades 7 through 12, 2010. April 6, 2011.

46  Surgeon General's Expert Panel on Prescription Drug Abuse in Youth: Prescription Monitoring Program Roles. U.S. Department of Health & Human Services presentation, March 29, 2011. Washington, DC.

47  The Partnership for a Drug-Free America. The Partnership Attitude Tracking Study (PATS) Teens in grades 7 through 12. May 16, 2006.

48  The National Center on Addiction and Substance Abuse at Columbia University. National Survey of American Attitudes on Substance Abuse CVI: Teens and Parents. Conducted by: QEV Analytics, Ltd. August 2011.

49  Knight JR. Preventing and Treating Rx Drug Abuse in Youth. Presentation to the Surgeon General's Expert Panel on Prescription Drug Abuse in Youth. U.S. Department of Health and Human Services presentation, March 29, 2011. Washington, DC.

50  American Academy of Pediatrics. *Periodic Survey of Fellows #31: Practices and Attitudes Toward Adolescent Drug Screening.* Elk Grove Village, IL: American Academy of Pediatrics, Division of Child Health Research; 1997.

51  The Partnership for a Drug-Free America. Time to Act! Look for Signs and Symptoms. Available at http:;//timetoact.www.drugfree.org/think-look-for-signs-.html. Accessed January 12, 2010.

# APPENDICES

# Appendix A
*Guidelines From the FSMB Model Policy for the Use of Controlled Substances for the Treatment of Pain*

The entire text of the FSMB Model Policy—including the Introduction and Section I: Preamble—is at http://www.fsmb.org/pdf/2004_grpol_Controlled_Substances.pdf

**SECTION II: GUIDELINES**
The Board has adopted the following criteria when evaluating the physician's treatment of pain, including the use of controlled substances:

**EVALUATION OF THE PATIENT**—A medical history and physical examination must be obtained, evaluated, and documented in the medical record. The medical record should document the nature and intensity of the pain, current and past treatments for pain, underlying or coexisting diseases or conditions, the effect of the pain on physical and psychological function, and history of substance abuse. The medical record also should document the presence of one or more recognized medical indications for the use of a controlled substance.

**TREATMENT PLAN**—The written treatment plan should state objectives that will be used to determine treatment success, such as pain relief and improved physical and psychosocial function, and should indicate if any further diagnostic evaluations or other treatments are planned. After treatment begins, the physician should adjust drug therapy to the individual medical needs of each patient. Other treatment modalities or a rehabilitation program may be necessary, depending on the etiology of the pain and the extent to which the pain is associated with physical and psychosocial impairment.

**INFORMED CONSENT AND AGREEMENT FOR TREATMENT**—The physician should discuss the risks and benefits of the use of controlled substances with the patient, persons designated by the patient, or with the patient's surrogate or guardian if the patient is without medical decision-making capacity. The patient should receive prescriptions from one physician and one pharmacy whenever possible. If the patient is at high risk for medication abuse or has a history of substance abuse, the physician should consider the use of a written agreement between physician and patient outlining patient responsibilities, including

- urine/serum medication levels screening when requested;
- number and frequency of all prescription refills; and
- reasons for which drug therapy may be discontinued (e.g., violation of agreement).

**PERIODIC REVIEW**—The physician should periodically review the course of pain treatment and any new information about the etiology of the pain or the patient's state of health. Continuation or modification of controlled substances for pain management therapy depends on the physician's evaluation of progress toward treatment objectives. Satisfactory response to treatment may be indicated by the patient's decreased pain, increased level of function, or improved quality of life. Objective evidence of improved or diminished function should be monitored and information from family members or other caregivers should be considered in determining the patient's response to treatment. If the patient's progress is unsatisfactory, the physician should assess the appropriateness of continued use of the current treatment plan and consider the use of other therapeutic modalities.

**CONSULTATION**—The physician should be willing to refer the patient as necessary for additional evaluation and treatment in order to achieve treatment objectives. Special attention should be given to those patients with pain who are at risk for medication misuse, abuse, or diversion. The management of pain in patients with a history of substance abuse or with a comorbid psychiatric disorder may require extra care, monitoring, documentation, and consultation with or referral to an expert in the management of such patients.

**MEDICAL RECORDS**—The physician should keep accurate and complete records to include

1. The medical history and physical examination,
2. Diagnostic, therapeutic and laboratory results,
3. Evaluations and consultations,
4. Treatment objectives,
5. Discussion of risks and benefits,
6. Informed consent,
7. Treatments,
8. Medications (including date, type, dosage and quantity prescribed),
9. Instructions and agreements, and
10. Periodic reviews.

Records should remain current and be maintained in an accessible manner and readily available for review.

**COMPLIANCE WITH CONTROLLED SUBSTANCES LAWS AND REGULATIONS**—To prescribe, dispense or administer controlled substances, the physician must be licensed in the state and comply with applicable federal and state regulations. Physicians are referred to the Physicians Manual of the U.S. Drug Enforcement Administration and (any relevant documents issued by the state medical board) for specific rules governing controlled substances as well as applicable state regulations.

# Appendix B
## APS-AAPM Clinical Guidelines

These Guidelines, published in 2009, resulted from the commissioning of an expert panel to review the evidence on chronic opioid therapy (COT) for chronic noncancer pain. Although evidence is limited, the panel concluded that chronic opioid therapy can be an effective therapy for carefully selected and monitored patients. The panel noted, however, that opioids are also associated with potentially serious harms, including opioid-related adverse effects and outcomes related to the abuse potential of opioids. Here is a summary of the panel's recommendations:

### PATIENT SELECTION AND RISK STRATIFICATION

- Before initiating COT, clinicians should conduct a history, physical examination and appropriate testing, including an assessment of risk of substance abuse, misuse, or addiction.

- Clinicians may consider a trial of COT as an option if chronic non-cancer pain (CNCP) is moderate or severe, pain is having an adverse impact on function or quality of life, and potential therapeutic benefits outweigh or are likely to outweigh potential harms.

- A benefit-to-harm evaluation including a history, physical examination, and appropriate diagnostic testing, should be performed and documented before and on an ongoing basis during COT.

### INFORMED CONSENT AND OPIOID MANAGEMENT PLANS

- When starting COT, informed consent should be obtained. A continuing discussion with the patient regarding COT should include goals, expectations, potential risks, and alternatives to COT.

- Clinicians may consider using a written COT management plan to document patient and clinician responsibilities and expectations and assist in patient education.

### INITIATION AND TITRATION OF CHRONIC OPIOID THERAPY

- Clinicians and patients should regard initial treatment with opioids as a therapeutic trial to determine whether COT is appropriate.

- Opioid selection, initial dosing, and titration should be individualized according to the patient's health status, previous exposure to opioids, attainment of therapeutic goals, and predicted or observed harms.

- There is insufficient evidence to recommend short-acting versus long-acting opioids, or as-needed versus around-the-clock dosing of opioids.

### METHADONE

- Methadone is characterized by complicated and variable pharmacokinetics and pharmacodynamics and should be initiated and titrated cautiously, by clinicians familiar with its use and risks.

### MONITORING

- Clinicians should reassess patients on COT periodically and as warranted by changing circumstances.

- Monitoring should include documentation of pain intensity and level of functioning, assessments of progress toward achieving therapeutic goals, presence of adverse events, and adherence to prescribed therapies.

- In patients on COT who are at high risk or who have engaged in aberrant drug-related behaviors, clinicians should periodically obtain urine drug screens or other information to confirm adherence to the COT plan of care.

- In patients on COT not at high risk and not known to have engaged in aberrant drug-related behaviors, clinicians should consider periodically obtaining urine drug screens or other information to confirm adherence to the COT plan of care.

### HIGH-RISK PATIENTS

- Clinicians may consider COT for patients with CNCP and history of drug abuse, psychiatric issues, or serious aberrant drug-related behaviors only if they are able to implement more frequent and stringent monitoring parameters. In such situations, clinicians should strongly consider consultation with a mental health or addiction specialist.

- Clinicians should evaluate patients engaging in aberrant drug-related behaviors for appropriateness of COT or need for restructuring of therapy, referral for assistance in management, or discontinuation of COT.

### DOSE ESCALATIONS, HIGH-DOSE OPIOID THERAPY, OPIOID ROTATION, AND INDICATIONS FOR DISCONTINUATION OF THERAPY

- When repeated dose escalations occur in patients on COT, clinicians should evaluate potential causes and reassess benefits relative to harms.

- In patients who require relatively high doses of COT, clinicians should evaluate for unique opioid-related adverse effects, changes in health status, and adherence to the COT treatment plan on an ongoing basis, and consider more frequent follow-up visits.

- Clinicians should consider opioid rotation when patients on COT experience intolerable adverse effects or inadequate benefit despite dose increases.

- Clinicians should taper or wean patients off of COT who engage in repeated aberrant drug-related behaviors or drug abuse/diversion, experience no progress toward meeting therapeutic goals, or experience intolerable adverse effects.

### OPIOID-RELATED ADVERSE EFFECTS

- Clinicians should anticipate, identify, and treat common opioid-associated adverse effects.

### USE OF PSYCHOTHERAPEUTIC COINTERVENTIONS

- As CNCP is often a complex biopsychosocial condition, clinicians who prescribe COT should routinely integrate psychotherapeutic interventions, functional restoration, interdisciplinary therapy, and other adjunctive nonopioid therapies.

### DRIVING AND WORK SAFETY

- Clinicians should counsel patients on COT about transient or lasting cognitive impairment that may affect driving and work safety. Patients should be counseled not to drive or engage in potentially dangerous activities when impaired or if they describe or demonstrate signs of impairment.

### IDENTIFYING A MEDICAL HOME AND WHEN TO OBTAIN CONSULTATION

- Patients on COT should identify a clinician who accepts primary responsibility for their overall medical care. This clinician may or may not prescribe COT, but should coordinate consultation and communication among all clinicians involved in the patient's care.

- Clinicians should pursue consultation, including interdisciplinary pain management, when patients with CNCP may benefit from additional skills or resources that they cannot provide.

### BREAKTHROUGH PAIN

- In patients on around-the-clock COT with breakthrough pain, clinicians may consider as-needed opioids based upon an initial and ongoing analysis of therapeutic benefit versus risk.

### OPIOIDS IN PREGNANCY

- Clinicians should counsel women of childbearing potential about the risks and benefits of COT during pregnancy and after delivery. Clinicians should encourage minimal or no use of COT during pregnancy, unless potential benefits outweigh risks. If COT is used during pregnancy, clinicians should be prepared to anticipate and manage risks to the patient and newborn.

### OPIOID POLICIES

- Clinicians should be aware of current federal and state laws, regulatory guidelines, and policy statements that govern the medical use of COT for CNCP.

# Appendix C
## *Additional Recent Guidance Documents*

Below is a list of recent guidelines or position statements related to opioid prescribing from professional groups and state or federal agencies from 2008 through 2012.

1. American Academy of Addiction Psychiatry (AAAP): Use of Opioids for the Treatment of Chronic, Nonmalignant Pain 2009 http://www2.aaap.org/sites/default/files/Use%20of%20Opioids %20in%20Chronic%20Pain%20Treatment%2C%202009. pdf?phpMyAdmin=H6N%2CWzwzCJE-qgHtALaDIa7GNj5

2. American College of Occupational and Environmental Medicine (ACOEM): Guidelines for the Chronic Use of Opioids 2011 http://www.acoem.org/uploadedFiles/Knowledge_Centers/ Practice_Guidelines/Chronic%20Pain%20Opioid%202011.pdf

3. American Geriatric Society (AGS): Pharmacological Management of Persistent Pain in Older Persons Guidelines (2009) http://www.americangeriatrics.org/health_care_professionals/ clinical_practice/clinical_guidelines_recommendations/2009/

4. American Pain Society / American Academy of Pain Medicine (APS/AAPM): Guideline for the Use of Chronic Opioid Therapy in Chronic Non-Cancer Pain - Evidence Review http://www.ampainsoc.org/library/pdf/Opioid_Final_Evidence_ Report.pdf

5. American Society of Anesthesiology / American Society of Regional Anesthesia and Pain Medicine: Practice Guidelines for Chronic Pain Management: An Updated Report by the American Society of Anesthesiologists Task Force on Chronic Pain Manage-

ment and the American Society of Regional Anesthesia and Pain Medicine 2010. http://journals.lww.com/anesthesiology/Full-text/2010/04000/Practice_Guidelines_for_Chronic_Pain_Management_.13.aspx

6. American Society of Interventional Pain Physicians (ASIPP): Opioids in the Management of Chronic Non-Cancer Pain: An Update of American Society of the Interventional Pain Physicians' (ASIPP) Guidelines 2008 http://www.painphysicianjournal.com/2008/march/2008;11;S5-S62.pdf

7. Collaborative National Opioid Use Guideline Group (NOUGG): Canadian Guideline for Safe and Effective Use of Opioids for Chronic Non-Cancer Part-A & B 2010 http://nationalpaincentre.mcmaster.ca/opioid/

8. Cochrane Collaboration Review: Long-Term Opioid Management for Chronic Non-Cancer Pain Review 2010 http://onlinelibrary.wiley.com/doi/10.1002/14651858.CD006605.pub2/pdf

9. Substance Abuse and Mental Health Services Administration TIP 54 (SAMHSA): Managing Chronic Pain in Adults With or in Recovery From Substance Use Disorders 2012 http://store.samhsa.gov/shin/content//SMA12-4671/SMA12-4671.pdf

10. Institute of Clinical Systems Improvement (ICSI): Health Care Guideline: Assessment and Management of Chronic Pain 2011 http://www.icsi.org/pain__chronic__assessment_and_management_of_14399/pain__chronic__assessment_and_management_of__guideline_.html

11. Institute of Medicine of the National Academies Pain Report, Relieving Pain in America A Blueprint for Transforming Prevention, Care, Education and Research 2011 http://www.iom.edu/~/media/Files/Report%20Files/2011/

Relieving-Pain-in-America-A-Blueprint-for-Transforming-
Prevention-Care-Education-Research/Pain%20Research%20
2011%20Report%20Brief.pdf

12. Maine Primary Care Association – Healthcare Safety Net Series:
    Opiate Use for Chronic, Non-Cancer Pain (CNCP) 2011
    http://www.mepca.org/Opiate_White_Paper.pdf

13. Office of National Drug Control Policy (ONDCP) Action Plan:
    Epidemic: Responding to America's prescription Drug Abuse
    Crisis 2011
    http://www.whitehouse.gov/sites/default/files/ondcp/issues-
    content/prescription-drugs/rx_abuse_plan.pdf

14. Physician's for Responsible Opioid Prescribing: Cautious,
    Evidence-Based Opioid Prescribing 2011
    http://www.supportprop.org/educational/PROP_
    OpioidPrescribing.pdf

15. Utah Department of Health: Utah Clinical Guidelines on
    Prescribing Opioids 2009
    http://www.dopl.utah.gov/licensing/forms/OpioidGuidlines.pdf

16. Veteran's Affairs / Department of Defense: Clinical Practice
    Guidelines: Summary Management of Opioid Therapy for
    Chronic Pain 2010
    http://www.healthquality.va.gov/COT_312_SUM-er.pdf

17. Washington State Guidelines: Interagency Guideline on Opioid
    Dosing for Chronic Non-Cancer Pain (CNCP) 2010
    http://www.agencymeddirectors.wa.gov/Files/OpioidGdline.pdf

18. World Health Organization: Ensuring Balance in National
    Policies on Controlled Substance 2011
    http://www.painpolicy.wisc.edu/publicat/11WHOGLs/
    WHOGLs.pdf

# Appendix D
## *Links to Pain Assessment Tools*

A variety of pain assessment tools is available on the website of the Federation of State Medical Boards in the Resource section: http://www.fsmb.org/pain-resources.html

In addition, here are links to four popular, well-validated pain assessment tools:

| Tool | URL |
|---|---|
| McGill Questionnaire | http://prc.coh.org/pdf/McGill%20Pain%20Questionnaire.pdf |
| Brief Pain Inventory (BPI) | medicine.iupui.edu/RHEU/Physicians/bpisf.pdf |
| Current Opioid Misuse Measure (COMM) | www.inflexxion.com/COMM |
| Pain Assessment and Documentation Tool (PADT) | www.healthinsight.org/Internal/assets/SMART/PADT.pdf |

# Appendix E
## *Dosing Thresholds for Selected Opioids*

| Opioid | Recommended dose threshold for seeking a pain consultation | Recommended starting dose for opioid-naive patients | Considerations |
|---|---|---|---|
| Codeine | 800mg per 24 hours | 30mg q 4-6 hours | • See individual product labeling for maximum dosing of combination products<br>• Avoid concurrent use of any OTC products containing same ingredient |
| Fentanyl transdermal | 50mcg/hour (q 72 hr) | N/A | • Use only in opioid-tolerant patients who have been taking ≥ 60mg MED daily for a week or longer |
| Hydrocodone | 30mg per 24 hours | 5-10mg q 4-6 hours | • See individual product labeling for maximum dosing of combination products<br>• Avoid concurrent use of any OTC products containing same ingredient |
| Hydromorphone | 30mg per 24 hours | 2mg q 4-6 hours | • Available in a more concentrated injectable solution (HP), intended for use only in opioid-tolerant patients |
| Morphine | 120mg per 24 hours | Immediate-release: 5 mg q 4-6 hours<br>Sustained-release: 10mg q 12 hours | • Adjust dose for renal impairment |
| Oxycodone | 80mg per 24 hours | Immediate-release: 5 mg q 4-6 hours<br>Sustained-release: 10mg q 12 hours | • See individual product labeling for maximum dosing of combination products<br>• Avoid concurrent use of any OTC products containing same ingredient |
| Oxymorphone | 40mg per 24 hours | Immediate-release: 5-10mg q 4-6 hours | • Use with extreme caution due to potential fatal interaction with alcohol or medications containing alcohol |

see Warnings and Recommendations on next page

**WARNINGS AND RECOMMENDATIONS**

- Hepatotoxicity can result from prolonged use or doses in excess of recommended maximum total daily dose of acetaminophen including over-the-counter products: short-term use (<10 days) = 4000 mg/day; long-term use = 2500mg/day.

- All conversions between opioids are estimates generally based on "equianalgesic dosing" or ED. Patient variability in response to these EDs can be large, due primarily to genetic factors and incomplete cross-tolerance. **It is recommended that, after calculating the appropriate conversion dose, it be reduced by 25–50% to assure patient safety.**

- Always monitor for adverse effects (nausea, constipation, over-sedation, itching, etc.)

- Prescribers must recognize that patients are complex and require individualized approaches that incorporate a rational protocol to carefully accomplish incremental steps based on safe timing intervals, dosing, and observation of patient responses.

- Caution must be used in converting from one opioid to another at any dose, and particularly at high doses.

- Opioid metabolism, mechanisms of action, and cross-tolerance may greatly differ between different opioid drugs. Conversion tables may be inaccurate for any given individual patient. Converting to or from methadone is particularly difficult and requires special care.

Source: Utah Department of Health, 2009. Adapted from Washington State Agency Medical Director's Group, 2007 and Webster, 2005

# Appendix F
## *Treatment Options for Opioid Side Effects*

**PREVENTING AND MANAGING SIDE EFFECTS**

| Side Effect | Prevention | Treatment |
| --- | --- | --- |
| Nausea | Co-prescribe antiemetic based on patient concomitant disease states and likelihood of adverse reactions or drug interactions | Antihistamines, antipsychotics, serotonin antagonists, prokinetic agents |
| Constipation | Prophylactic treatments including increase fluid and fiber intake, increased exercise, stimulant laxatives, osmotic agents, bulk-forming laxatives. | Periodic use of saline laxatives or administration of suppositories or enemas. Consider transdermal fentanyl. |
| Impaired cognition | For high-risk (e.g., Alzheimer's) patients maximize non-opioid regimen | Lower dose; rotate to another opioid; low-dose neuroleptics if necessary |
| Pruritus | Probability of pruritus is increased with epidural or intraspinal administration. | Rotate to another opioid; reduce dose; antihistamines; consider paroxetine |
| Rash/hives | If patient has history, use opioid in different chemical group or family | Rotate to another opioid; symptomatic treatment |
| Respiratory depression | "Start low, go slow." Start with low doses of opioid and titrate to effect; monitor patient closely | Close observation, supportive measures (airway, breathing, and circulation, or "ABC"); naloxone for overdose with respiratory or hemodynamic compromise |
| Sedation | "Start low, go slow." Start with low doses of opioid and titrate to effect; monitor patient closely | Lower dose; add co-analgesics; add stimulants |
| Myoclonus | N/A | Rotate to another opioid; consider low doses of baclofen, clonazepam, or gabapentin |

Adapted from: Swegle JM, Logemann C. *American Family Physician.* 2006 Oct 15;74(8):1347-1354.

# Appendix G
## *Medicines Recommended for Disposal by Flushing*

The Food and Drug Administration (FDA) recommends that the following expired, unwanted, or unused medicines be flushed down a sink or toilet to help prevent misuse or diversion. This list was revised in March 2010. For more recent updates, check: www.fda.gov/Drugs/ResourcesForYou/Consumers.

*(Note: Some states and municipalities may have different or more stringent guidelines.)*

| Medicine | Active Ingredient |
|---|---|
| **Actiq**, oral transmucosal lozenge * | Fentanyl Citrate |
| **Avinza**, capsules (extended release) | Morphine Sulfate |
| **Daytrana**, transdermal patch system | Methylphenidate |
| **Demerol**, tablets * | Meperidine Hydrochloride |
| **Demerol**, oral solution * | Meperidine Hydrochloride |
| **Diastat/Diastat AcuDial**, rectal gel | Diazepam |
| **Dilaudid**, tablets * | Hydromorphone Hydrochloride |
| **Dilaudid**, oral liquid * | Hydromorphone Hydrochloride |
| **Dolophine Hydrochloride**, tablets * | Methadone Hydrochloride |
| **Duragesic**, patch (extended release) * | Fentanyl |
| **Embeda**, capsules (extended release) | Morphine Sulfate; Naltrexone Hydrochloride |
| **Exalgo**, tablets (extended release) | Hydromorphone Hydrochloride |
| **Fentora**, tablets (buccal) | Fentanyl Citrate |
| **Kadian**, capsules (extended release) | Morphine Sulfate |
| **Methadone Hydrochloride**, oral solution * | Methadone Hydrochloride |
| **Methadose**, tablets * | Methadone Hydrochloride |
| **Morphine Sulfate**, tablets (immediate release) * | Morphine Sulfate |

| Morphine Sulfate, oral solution * | Morphine Sulfate |
|---|---|
| MS Contin, tablets (extended release) * | Morphine Sulfate |
| Onsolis, soluble film (buccal) | Fentanyl Citrate |
| Opana, tablets (immediate release) | Oxymorphone Hydrochloride |
| Opana ER, tablets (extended release) | Oxymorphone Hydrochloride |
| Oramorph SR, tablets (sustained release) | Morphine Sulfate |
| Oxycontin, tablets (extended release) * | Oxycodone Hydrochloride |
| Percocet, tablets * | Acetaminophen; Oxycodone Hydrochloride |
| Percodan, tablets * | Aspirin; Oxycodone Hydrochloride |
| Xyrem, oral solution | Sodium Oxybate |

*These medicines have generic versions available or are only available in generic formulations.

# About the Author

Scott M. Fishman, M.D., is a nationally recognized author and advocate for patients in pain. He is Chief of the Division of Pain Medicine and Professor of Anesthesiology and Pain Medicine at the University of California, Davis. He was formerly Medical Director of the Massachusetts General Hospital Pain Center at Harvard Medical School. Dr. Fishman completed residency training in Internal Medicine at Greenwich Hospital and Yale University School of Medicine, and Psychiatry residency at Massachusetts General Hospital and Harvard Medical School. He completed his pain fellowship in the Department of Anesthesia of Massachusetts General Hospital and Harvard Medical School. He has been board certified in Internal Medicine, Psychiatry, Pain Medicine, and Hospice and Palliative Care.

Dr. Fishman is the author of *The War on Pain* (HarperCollins) and *Listening to Pain* (Oxford University Press), and the co-author *Spinal Cord Stimulation: Implantation Techniques* (Oxford University Press). He has also co-edited *Bonica's Management of Pain* 4th edition (Lippincott), *Essentials of Pain Medicine and Regional Anesthesia* (Elsevier), and *The Massachusetts General Hospital Handbook of Pain Management* 2nd edition (Lippincott). He has authored many peer-reviewed articles in medical journals, book chapters, and other scholarly reviews. He serves as Senior Editor for the journal Pain Medicine and sits on the editorial board of other medical journals.

Dr. Fishman is Past President of the American Academy of Pain Medicine, Past Chair of the Board of the American Pain Foundation, and has served on the board of directors of the American Pain Society. He has helped national and state legislatures with pain-related laws and consults to numerous state and federal government agencies.